TABLE OF CONTENTS

TOP 20 TEST TAKING TIPS ....

MICROBIOLOGY REVIEW 8
    CHARACTERISTICS OF BACTERIA TYPES 8
    IMMUNOGLOBULIN ISOTYPES 11
    CYTOKINES REVIEW 11
    DENTAL DECAY 11

GENERAL MEDICAL PATHOLOGICAL CONDITIONS 14
    DISORDERS OF THE EYE 16
    DISORDERS OF THE EAR 18

DENTISTRY RELATED PATHOLOGICAL CONDITIONS 19
    RED LESIONS 19
    WHITE LESIONS 22
    TMJ REVIEW 27

MAJOR FUNCTIONS OF CELLS MEDIATING IMMUNE RESPONSES 29

ANATOMIC SCIENCES 30

AXIAL SKELETON 30

APPENDICULAR SKELETON 30

FOUR BASIC TISSUES 34

INTEGUMENTARY (SKIN) SYSTEM 37

MUSCLES OF MASTICATION 39

MUSCLES OF EXPRESSION 40

NEUROLOGY REVIEW 40
    BRAIN 40

SPINAL TRACTS 47
    BASAL GANGLIA REVIEW 50

RESPIRATORY/CARDIAC REVIEW 51

RESPIRATORY CONDITIONS 53

CIRCULATORY SYSTEM 55
Course of Circulation 55
The Heart 56
Cardiovascular Conditions 58

ENDOCRINE REVIEW 59

GENETICS AND CELL BIOLOGY 61
The Cell- Its Structures and Function 62
Composition of Protoplasm 63
Components of a typical Cell 65
Mitochondria 67
Endoplasmic Reticulum (ER) 69
Lysosome 69
Nucleus 70
Cell Division – Mitosis 72
Polygenic Traits 73
Major Hormones 74
Gland Review 75

DENTAL ANATOMY 76
Key Terms 76
The Basics 77
Jaws and Dental Arches 78
Classes of Teeth 80
Dental Formula, Dental Notation, Universal Numbering System 81
Parts of the Tooth 82
Dental Tissues 82
Points of Reference 83
Dental Terminology 83
Location and position 85
Teeth 86
COMPARISON OF TISSUES OF THE TEETH 88

- Investing Structures ... 89
- Deciduous Dentition ... 91
- The Transition from the Deciduous to the Permanent Dentition ... 92
- Deciduous Dentition ... 93
- Summary ... 94

OCCLUSION ... 95

- (Stages of dentofacial development) ... 95
- Permanent dentition period ... 98
- Curve of Spee ... 99
- Overjet and overbite ... 99
- Compensating curvatures of the individual teeth ... 100
- Normal or 'Ideal' Occlusion ... 100
- Age and Aging of Teeth ... 105
- The Permanent Incisor Teeth ... 106
- The Permanent Canine Teeth ... 110
- The Premolar Teeth ... 112
- Caries ... 124
- Sealants ... 127
- Dental Emergencies and Treatment ... 129

SECRET KEY #1 - TIME IS YOUR GREATEST ENEMY ... 130

- Pace Yourself ... 130

SECRET KEY #2 - GUESSING IS NOT GUESSWORK ... 131

- Monkeys Take the Test ... 131
- $5 Challenge ... 131

SECRET KEY #3 - PRACTICE SMARTER, NOT HARDER ... 133

- Success Strategy ... 133

SECRET KEY #4 - PREPARE, DON'T PROCRASTINATE ... 134

SECRET KEY #5 - TEST YOURSELF ... 135

GENERAL STRATEGIES ... 136

- Be Aware of the Following Hints ... 141
- Registering for the NBDE Part I Licensure Test ... 141

NBDE Part I Score Reporting 142

SPECIAL REPORT- STUDY GUIDES AND PRACTICE TESTS ARE WORTH YOUR TIME 143
Practice Questions 143
Study Guides 143

SPECIAL REPORT- QUICK REFERENCE LESION REVIEW 144

SPECIAL REPORT- REVIEW TABLES AND IMAGES 145

CPR REVIEW/CHEAT SHEET 154
Conscious Choking 154
Unconscious Choking 154
Rescue Breaths 154

AED 154

SPECIAL REPORT: ADDITIONAL BONUS MATERIAL 155

Top 20 Test Taking Tips

1. Carefully follow all the test registration procedures
2. Know the test directions, duration, topics, question types, how many questions
3. Setup a flexible study schedule at least 3-4 weeks before test day
4. Study during the time of day you are most alert, relaxed, and stress free
5. Maximize your learning style; visual learner use visual study aids, auditory learner use auditory study aids
6. Focus on your weakest knowledge base
7. Find a study partner to review with and help clarify questions
8. Practice, practice, practice
9. Get a good night's sleep; don't try to cram the night before the test
10. Eat a well balanced meal
11. Know the exact physical location of the testing site; drive the route to the site prior to test day
12. Bring a set of ear plugs; the testing center could be noisy
13. Wear comfortable, loose fitting, layered clothing to the testing center; prepare for it to be either cold or hot during the test
14. Bring at least 2 current forms of ID to the testing center
15. Arrive to the test early; be prepared to wait and be patient
16. Eliminate the obviously wrong answer choices, then guess the first remaining choice
17. Pace yourself; don't rush, but keep working and move on if you get stuck
18. Maintain a positive attitude even if the test is going poorly
19. Keep your first answer unless you are positive it is wrong
20. Check your work, don't make a careless mistake

Microbiology Review

Characteristics of Bacteria Types

Rickettsias- gram-negative bacteria, small
Rickettsia rickettsii

Spirochetes- spiral shape, no flagella, slender
Lyme disease, Treponema pallidum-syphilis

Gram positive cocci- Hold color with Gram stain, ovoid or spherical shape
Staphlyococcus aureus, Streptococcus pneumoniae

Gram negative cocci- Loose color with Gram stain, spherical or oval shape
Neisseria meningidis (meningococcus), *Neisseria gonorrhoeae* (gonococcus)

Mycoplasmas- *Mycoplasma pneumoniae*

Acid-fast bacilli- Hold color with staining even when stained with acid in most cases. *Mycobacterium leprae, Mycobacterium tuberculosis*

Acitinomycetes- Stained positive with a gram stain, narrow filaments
Nocardia, Actinomyces israelii

Gram positive- Rod shaped, hold color with gram stain
Clostridium tetani, Bacillus anthracis

Gram negative- Do not hold color with gram stain, also rod shaped.
Pseudomonas aeruginosa, Escherichia coli, Klebsiella pneumoniae

Diseases and Acid Fast Bacilli Review

Disease	Bacteria	Primary Medication
Tuberculosis, renal and meningeal infections	*Mycobacterium tuberculosis*	Isoniazid + rifampin + pyrazinamide
Leprosy	*Mycobacterium leprae*	Dapsone + rifampin

Diseases and Spirochetes Review

Disease	Bacteria	Primary Medication
Lyme Disease	*Borrelia burgdorferi*	Tetracycline
Meningitis	*Leptospira*	Penicillin G

| Syphilis | *Treponema pallidum* | Penicillin G |

Diseases and Actinomycetes Review

Disease	Bacteria	Primary Medication
Cervicofacial, and other lesions	*Actinomyces israelii*	Penicillin G

Diseases and Gram-Negative Bacilli Review

Disease	Bacteria	Primary Medication
Meningitis	*Flavobacterium meningosepticum*	Vancomycin
UTI's Bacteremia	*Escherichia coli*	Ampicillin+/- aminoglycoside
Gingivitis, Genital infections, ulcerative pharyngitis	*Fusobacterium nucleatum*	Penicillin G
Abscesses	*Bacteroides species*	Clindamycin/Penicillin G
Hospital acquired infections	*Acinetobacter*	Aminoglycoside
Abscesses, Endocarditis	*Bacteroides fragilis*	Clindamycin, metronidazole
Legionnaires' Disease	*Legionella pneumonphila*	Erythromycin
UTI's	*Proteus mirabilis*	Ampicillin/Amoxicillin
Pneumonia, UTI's, Bacteremia	*Pseudomonas aeruginosa*	Penicillin-Broad
Bacteremia, Endocarditis	*Streptobacillus moniliformis*	Penicillin G
Pneumonia, UTI	*Klebsiella pneumoniae*	Cephalosporin
Bacteremia, Wound infections	*Pasteurella multocida*	Penicillin G

Diseases and Gram-Positive Bacilli Review

Disease	Bacteria	Primary Medication
Gas Gangrene	*Clostridium*	Penicillin G
Tetanus	*Clostridium tetani*	Penicillin G
Pharyngitis	*Corynebacterium diphtheriae*	Penicillin G
Meningitis, Bacteremia	*Listeria monocytogenes*	Ampicillin

| Anthrax / pneumonia | *Bacillus anthracis* | Penicillin G |
| Endocarditis | *Corynebacterium species* | Penicillin G/Vancomycin |

Diseases and Cocci Review

Disease	Bacteria	Primary Medication
Genital infections, arthritis-dermatitis syndrome	*Neisseria gonorrhoeae*	Ampicillin, Amoxicillin
Meningitis, Bacteremia	*Neisseria meningitidis*	Penicillin G
Endocarditis, Bacteremia	*Streptococcus (viridans group)*	Gentamicin
Bacteremia, brain and other absesses	*Streptococcus (anaerobic species)*	Penicillin G
Endocarditis, Bacteremia	*Streptococcus agalactiae*	Ampicillin
Pneumonia, Osteomyelitis, abscesses	*Staphyloccus aureus*	Penicillin G/Vancomycin
UTI's, Endocarditis	*Streptococcus faecalis*	Ampicillin, Penicillin G
Pneumonia, sinusitis, otitis, Arthritis	*Streptococcus pneumoniae*	Penicillin G or V
Cellulitis, Scarlet fever, bacteremia	*Streptococcus pyogenes*	Penicillin G or V
Bacteremia, endocarditis	*Streptococcus bovis*	Penicillin G

DNA Virus Review

DNA Virus	*Infection*
Adenovirus	Eye and Respiratory infections
Hepatitis B	Hepatitis B
Cytomegalovirus	Cytomegalic inclusion disease
Epstein-Barr	Infectious mononucleosis
Herpes Types 1 and 2	Local infections oral and genital
Varicella-zoster	Chickenpox, herpes zoster
Smallpox	Smallpox

RNA Virus Review

RNA Virus	*Infection*
Human respiratory virus	Respiratory tract infection
Hepatitis A virus	Hepatitis A
Influenza virus A-C	Influenza
Measles virus	Measles
Mumps virus	Mumps

Respiratory syncytial virus	Respiratory tract infection in children
Poliovirus	Poliomyelitis
Rhinovirus types 1-89	Cold
Human immunodeficiency virus	AIDS
Rabies virus	Rabies
Alphavirus	Encephalitis
Rubella virus	Rubella

Immunoglobulin isotypes

IgA– can be located in secretions and prevents viral and bacterial attachment to membranes.
IgD- can be located on B cells
IgE-main mediator of mast cells with allergen exposure.
IgG- primarily found in secondary responses. Does cross placenta and destroys viruses/bacteria.
IgM- primarily found in first response. Located on B cells

Cytokines Review

IL-1   Primarily stimulate of fever response. Helps activate B and T cells. Produced by macrophages.
IL-2   Aids in the development of Cytotoxic T cells and helper cells. Produced by helper T cells.
IL-3   Aids in the development of bone marrow stem cells. Produced by T-cells.
IL-4   Aids in the growth of B cells. Produced by helper T-cells. Aids in the production of IgG and IgE
IL-5   Promotes the growth of eosinophils. Produced by helper T-cells. Also promotes IgA production.
IL-8   Neutrophil factor
TNF-α Promotes the activation of neutrophils and is produced by macrophages.
TNF-β Produced by T lymphocytes and encourages the activation of neutrophils
γ-interferon   (Activates macrophages and is produced by helper T cells.)

Dental Decay

Dental decay is due to the irreversible solubilization of tooth mineral by acid produced by certain bacteria that adhere to the tooth surface in bacterial communities known as dental plaque.

Streptococcus mutans is the main cause of dental decay. Various lactobacilli are associated with progression of the lesion.

Pathogenesis
The tooth surface normally loses some tooth mineral from the action of the acid formed by plaque bacteria after ingestion of foods containing fermentable carbohydrates. This mineral is normally replenished by the saliva between meals. However, when fermentable foods are eaten frequently, the low pH in the plaque is sustained and a net loss of mineral from the tooth occurs. This low pH selects for aciduric organisms, such as *S mutans* and lactobacilli, which (especially *S mutans*) store polysaccharide and continue to secrete acid long after the food has been swallowed.

Clinical Manifestations
Caries become intensely painful when the lesion approaches the tooth pulp.

Microbiologic Diagnosis
New, chair-side culture procedures allow for an estimate of the number of *S mutans* organisms in saliva.

Periodontal Disease
Periodontal infections are usually mixed, most often involving anaerobes such as *Treponema denticola* and *Porphyromonas gingivalis*. The microaerophile *Actinobacillus actinomycetemcomitans* causes a rare form known as localized juvenile periodontitis.

Pathogenesis
Plaque bacteria elaborate various compounds (H2S, NH3, amines, toxins, enzymes, antigens, etc.) that elicit an inflammatory response that is protective but also is responsible for loss of periodontal tissue, pocket formation, and loosening and loss of teeth.
Clinical Manifestations
There is no apparent pain until very late when abscesses may occur. Bleeding gums and bad breath may occur.
Microbiologic Diagnosis
Microbiologic diagnosis is usually not sought. Spirochetes and other motile organisms are found upon dark-field microscopic examination. Immunologic reagents, DNA probes and enzyme assays have been developed for *P gingivalis, T denticola, Bacteroides forsythus, A actinomycetemcomitans* and other organisms.

Etiology
Dental decay has been known since recorded history, but was not an important health problem until sucrose became a major component of the human diet. When sucrose is consumed frequently, an organism known as *Streptococcus mutans*

emerges as the predominant organism, and it is this organism that has been uniquely associated with dental decay.

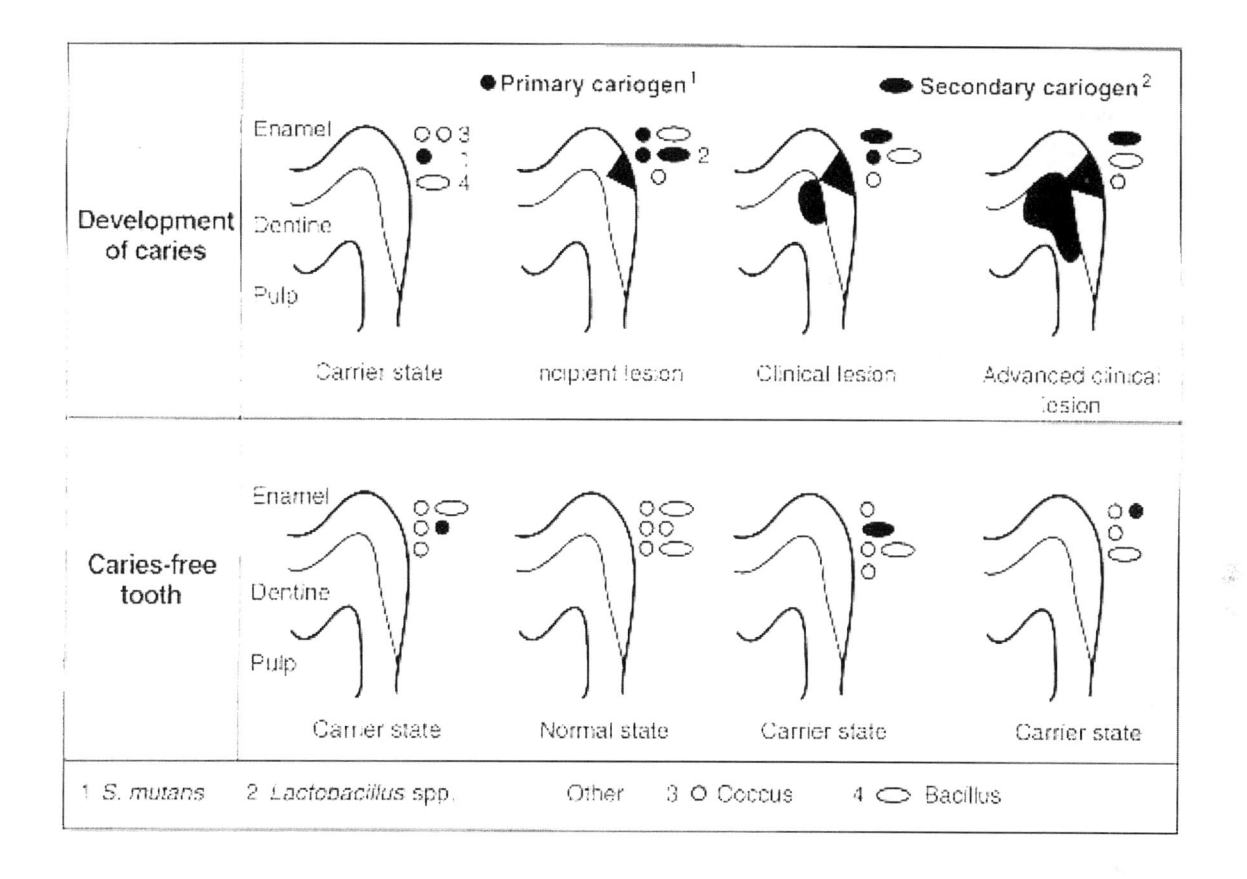

Development of caries	Carrier state	Incipient lesion	Clinical lesion	Advanced clinical lesion
Caries-free tooth	Carrier state	Normal state	Carrier state	Carrier state

1. *S. mutans* 2. *Lactobacillus* spp. Other 3. ○ Coccus 4. ⬭ Bacillus

● Primary cariogen [1]   ⬬ Secondary cariogen [2]

General Medical Pathological Conditions

1. AIDS- caused by a retrovirus in which viral RNA becomes part of the host cell DNA. Reduction in T-cells (<250) and a high viral load can cause HIV to progress to AIDS. Low immunity can lead to opportunistic infections like pneumoncystsis carinnii, secondary cancers, salmonella, neuropathies, and meningitis. Use of protease inhibitors in combination with other drugs seems to be a major step in the management of HIV.
2. Budd-Chiari syndrome- leads to congestive liver disease. Caused by an occlusion of the hepatic veins or IVC.
3. Cellulitis- inflammation of the connective tissue, tends to be widespread and is poorly defined. It is frequently accompanied by infection. The skin over the area is often hot, red, and edematous, and resembles the skin of an orange.
4. CHF- may result in tachycardia, decreased stroke volume, LE swelling and decreased cardiac output.
5. Cri-du-chat syndrome – Noted severe mental deficits and chromosome 5 short arm.
6. Cystic fibrosis – thickening of secretions of all exocrine glands, leading to obstruction. Probable multiple frequent respiratory infections especially Staph. Aureus and Pseudomonas Aeruginosa
7. Dermatitis- superficial inflammation of the skin, characterized by vesicles (when acute), redness, edema, oozing, crusting, scaling and usually itching
8. Deep vein thrombosis – formation of an abnormal blood clot in a deep vein. If the clot breaks free it may become a pulmonary embolus. Symptoms include a +Homan's sign, positive doppler. Anticoagulant therapy is indicated in most cases.
9. Diabetes Mellitus-Insulin dependent is due to the absolute insulin deficiency and can lead to diabetic ketoacidosis
10. Diabetes mellitus-non-insulin-dependent diabetes is usually associated with obesity and is caused by a combination of insulin resistance and a defect in beta-cell responsiveness to elevated plasma glucose concentration. Plasma insulin concentration is usually normal or elevated.
11. Fragile X syndrome- X-linked disease with appearance of enlarged testes, autism and enlarged jaw.
12. Down's syndrome- Trisomy 21-altered facial appearance, mental retardation, simian crease, congenital heart disease.
13. Duchenne's muscular dystrophy- X-linked recessive disease with noted pelvic weakness and calf hypertrophy.
14. Edward's syndrome- Trisomy 18- mental retardation, congenital heart disease, life span < 1 yr.
15. Eisenmenger's syndrome- Late cynosis due to increasing pulmonary hypertension.
16. Gout – metabolic disease marked by elevated level of serum uric acid and deposition of urate crystals in the joints, soft tissue and kidneys. Treatment

often involves anti-inflammatory medications, daily use of colchicine and lowering of urate concentration in body fluids with diet.
17. Hemophilia – bleeding disorder that is inherited and has to do with clotting factor deficiency.
18. Hepatitis – inflammation of the liver and may be caused by viral or bacterial infections or chemical agents. Transmission is from blood, body fluids, or body tissues, through oral or sexual contact or contaminated needles. Signs/Symptoms include elevated lab values of hepatic transaminases and bilirubin, enlarged liver with tenderness, fever and jaundice. Treatment-IV fluids, analgesics, interferon and vaccines
19. Herpes zoster – acute nervous system viral infection involving the dorsal root ganglia and characterized by vesicular eruption and neuralgic pain I the cutaneous areas supplied by peripheral sensory nerves arising at the infected dermatome or myotome. Treatment involves corticosteroids for pain relief in many cases.
20. Intermittent claudication – arterial insufficiency that results in ischemia to the exercising muscle. Relief of pain is achieved by resting.
21. Kartagener's syndrome-linked to situs inversus, causes sterility.
22. Lyme disease – inflammatory disease caused by a spirochete transmitted to humans by a tick bit and is common in the northeastern U. S. Treatment often involves antibiotic, medications for pain relief.
23. Paget's disease – slowly progressive metabolic bone disease characterized by an initial phase of excessive bone re-absorption followed by a reactive phase of excessive abnormal bone formation. The disease can be fatal when associated with CHF, bone sarcoma or giant cell tumors
24. Psoriasis – chronic disease of the skin with erythematous plaques covered with a silvery scale. Common on the scalp, elbows, knees, and genitalia. Treatment involves long-wave UV light, combination UV light with oral photosensitizing drug (Psoralen).
25. Pulmonary embolism- a thrombus from the peripheral venous circulation lodges in the pulmonary artery with the subsequent obstruction of blood flow to the lungs. Treatment often involves a low-dose heparin, analgesis, and pulmonary vasodilators.
26. Rhematoid arthritis – Complaints of fatigue, weight loss, weakness and general diffuse musculoskeletal pain are often the initial presentations. Pain is localized to specific joints with symmetrical bilateral presentation. Deformities of the fingers are common.
27. Reye's syndrome- (hepatoencephalophathy), sometimes fatal with children related to viruses and aspirin.
28. Systemic lupus erythematosus – chronic, systemic rheumatic, inflammatory disorder of the connective tissues which affects multiple organs including skin and joints.
29. Turner syndrome- Noted webbing of the neck and ovarian dysgenesis. (X0)
30. Tuberculosis – infection spread by droplets from the untreated infected host. Treatment involves medications to eliminate infection.

31. Wilson's Disease- (hepatolenticular degeneration) copper does not enter circulation and builds up in the brain, liver and eye.

Disorders of the Eye

Diabetic retinopathy:

Blood vessels in the retina are affected. Can lead to blindness if untreated. Two primary stages (Proliferative and Nonproliferative. Retina may experience bleeding in nonproliferative stage. During the proliferative stage damage begins moving towards the center of the eye and there is an increase in bleeding. Any damage caused is non-reversible. Only further damage can be prevented.

Strabismus: 斜視

Eyes are moving in different stages. The axes of the eyes are not parallel. Normally, treated with an eyepatch; however, eye drops are now used in many cases. Atropine drops are placed in the stronger eye for correction purposes. Surgery may be necessary in some cases. Suture surgery will reduce the pull of certain eye muscles.

Macular Degeneration: 黃斑部病變

Impaired central vision caused by destruction of the macula, which is the center part of the retina. Limited vision straight ahead. More common in people over 60. Can be characterized as dry or wet types. Wet type more common. Vitamin C, Zinc, and Vitamin E may help slow progression.

Esotropia: 內斜視

Appearance of cross-eyed gaze or internal strabismus.

Exotropia:

External strabismus or divergent gaze.

Conjunctivitis: 結膜炎

Inflammation of the conjuctiva, that can be caused by viruses or bacteria. Also known as pink eye. If viral source can be highly contagious. Antibiotic eye drops and warm cloths to the eye helpful treatment. Conjunctivitis can also be caused by chemicals or allergic reactions. Re-occurring conjunctivitis can indicate a larger underlying disease process.

Glaucoma: 青光眼

An increase in fluid pressure in the eye leading to possible optic nerve damage. More common in African-Americans. Minimal onset symptoms, often picked to late. Certain drugs may decrease the amount of fluid entering the eye. Two major types of glaucoma are open-angle glaucoma and angle-closure glaucoma.

Disorders of the Ear

Otitis media: 中耳炎

Most common caused by the bacteria (H.flu) and Streptococcus pneumoniae in about 85% of cases. 15% of cases viral related. More common in bottlefeeding babies. Can be caused by upper respiratory infections. Ear drums can rupture in severe cases. A myringotomy may be performed in severe cases to relieve pus in the middle ear.

Barotitis: 氣壓耳炎

Atmospheric pressures causing middle ear dysfunction. Any change in altitude causes problems.

Mastoiditis: 乳突炎

May be caused by an ear infection and is known as inflammation of the mastoid.

Meniere's disease:

Inner ear disorder. Causes unknown. Episodic rotational vertigo, Tinnitus, 耳鳴 Hearing loss, and Ringing in the ears are key symptoms. Dazide is the primary medication for Meniere's disease. Low salt diet and surgery are also other treatment options. Diagnosis is a rule-out diagnosis.

Labyrinthitis: 內耳迷路炎

Vertigo associated with nausea and malaise. Related to bacterial and viral infections. Inflammation of the labyrinth in the inner ear.

Otitis externa:

Usually caused by a bacterial infection. Swimmer's ear. Infection of the skin with the outer ear canal that progress to the ear drum. Itching, Drainage and Pain are the key symptoms. Suctioning of the ear canal may be necessary. Most common ear drops (Volsol, Cipro, Cortisporin).

Dentistry Related Pathological Conditions

Ludwig's Angina
Poor dental hygiene
Polymicrobial with streptococcus, staphylococcus and Bacteroides species predominating
Clinically, patients are toxic appearing and have "brawny" or "woody" induration of the neck above the hyoid bone It starts as a cellulitis but may progress to abscess.

ANUG
Acute necrotizing ulcerative gingivitis
Caused by infection of the gums with Fusobacteria and spirochetes
Risk factors are stress, smoking, poor dental hygiene

Red Lesions

Red lesions are a large group of disorders of the oral mucosa. Traumatic lesions, infections, developmental anomalies, allergic reactions, premalignant lesions, malignancies, and systemic disease are included in this group. The red color of the tissue may be due to thin epithelium (skin), inflammation, dilation of blood vessels or an increased number of blood vessels.

Types of Red Lesions

Traumatic erythema	Erythroplakia
Thermal burn	Contact allergic stomatitis
Geographic tongue	Hemangioma
Median Rhomboid glossitis	Lupus erythematous
Denture stomatitis	Anemia
Squamous-cell carcinoma	

Traumatic Erythema
The condition occurs when a traumatic event results in hemorrhage within the oral tissues.
Clinical features - Traumatic erythema can present as an ecchymosis (multiple small bruises) or a hematoma (a single larger bruise). Clinically, it appears as an irregular, usually flat, area with a bright or deep red color. The tongue, the lips, and the inside surfaces of the cheeks are the most common areas affected. Diagnosis is based on clinical appearance and patient history.
Treatment - None required.

Thermal Burn
Thermal burns to the oral mucosa are relatively common, usually due to contact with very hot foods and liquids.
Clinical features - The condition appears as a red, painful area that may undergo desquamation (peeling away of superficial layer of skin), leaving erosions. The lesions heal spontaneously in about a week.
Treatment - None required.

Geographic Tongue
Geographic tongue presents as multiple, well-defined patches of redness surrounded by a thin, raised whitish border. Usually, the lesions persist for a short time in one area, disappear within a few days, and then develop in another area. The top surface (dorsum) of the tongue is the most common area of development.

Treatment - None required.
Top of Page

Median Rhomboid Glossitis
Median rhomboid glossitis is a relatively rare condition that only occurs on the top surface of the tongue.
Cause - Believed to be developmental, though Candida albicans is also thought to play a role.
Clinical features - The condition presents as a well-demarcated red rhomboid-shaped area along the middle of the top surface of the tongue. The surface of the lesion may be smooth or lobulated.
Treatment - None required.

Denture Stomatitis
Denture stomatits, or sore mouth, is a frequent condition in patients who wear dentures continuously or for long periods of time.
Cause - Mechanical irritation from the dentures, candida albicans, or a tissue response to microorganisms living beneath the dentures.
Clinical features - The condition is characterized by diffuse redness, swelling (edema), occasionally bruising (petechiae) and white spots that represent accumulations of candidal hyphae. The condition is almost always located in the denture-bearing area of the maxilla (palate). The condition is usually asymptomatic.
Treatment - Improvement of denture fit , oral hygiene, and topical antimycotics.

Squamous Cell Carcinoma
The early stage of squamous cell carcinoma may present as an asymptomatic, atypical red patch. The clinical features are identical to erythroplakia. In these early stage, a biopsy should be taken to confirm diagnosis. For more information on squamous cell carcinoma, see our section on oral cancer.

Erythroplakia
The condition is defined as a red, nonspecific patch or plaque that cannot be classified as any other disease.
Cause - unknown
Clinical features - It appears asymptotically as a fiery red, demarcated plaque with a smooth and velvety surface. The floor of the mouth, soft palate area, and tongue are the most common sites of involvement. It occurs most frequently between the ages of 50 and 70. Over 91% of erythroplakias histologically demonstrate early invasive squamous-cell carcinoma at the time of diagnosis.
Treatment - surgical excision.

Contact Allergic Stomatitis
The condition is a rare acute or chronic allergic reaction.
Cause - Denture based materials, restorative materials, mouthwashes, toothpastes, foods, chewing gums, and other substances may be responsible.
Clinical features - The affected mucosa presents with diffuse redness and swelling and occasionally small vesicles and erosions. A burning sensation is a common symptom. In the chronic form, white lesions may be seen in addition to redness.
Laboratory tests - mucosal and skin patch tests.
Treatment - Removal of suspected allergens, topical or systemic steroids, antihistamines.

Hemangioma
The condition is a relatively common benign proliferation of blood vessels that primarily develops during childhood.
Cause - Developmental
Clinical features - Two main forms of the condition are recognized - capillary and cavernous. The capillary form presents as a flat red area consisting of numerous small capillaries. Cavernous hemangioma appears as an elevated lesion of a deep red color, and consists of large diluted sinuses filled with blood. A characteristic sign of hemangioma is that the red color disappears on pressure, and returns when the pressure is released.
Treatment - Surgical excision, cryotherapy, or laser.

Lupus Erythematous
The condition is a chronic immunologically mediated disease.
Clinical features - Two main forms of the disease are recognized - discoid and systemic. The oral lesions are characterized by a well-defined central red area surrounded by a sharp elevated border of irradiating whitish striae.
Laboratory tests - direct immunofluorescence, histopathological examination.
Treatment - steroids, antimalarials.

Anemia
Oral manifestations of anemia are early and common and are characterized by a

smooth, red tongue. a burning sensation, taste loss, angular chelitis (chaffing at the corners of the mouth) may also be noted.

White Lesions

White lesions of the oral mucosa are a multifactorial group of disorders, the colorof which is produced by the scattering of light through an altered epithelial (mucosal/ gum, tissue) surface.

Leukoplakia	Hairy tongue
Hairy Leukoplakia	Furred tongue
Lichen Planus	Materia alba of the gingiva
Linea Alba	Fordyce's granules
Nicotine Stomatitis	Leukoedema
Chemical burn	White spongy nevus
Candidiasis	Papilloma
Chronic Bitting	Verrucous carcinoma
Geographic tongue	Squamous-cell carcinoma

Leukoplakia
Leukoplakia is a clinical term. The lesion is defined as a white patch or plaque, firmly attached to the oral mucosa, that cannot be classified as any other disease. It is a pre-cancerous lesion.
Cause - The exact etiology or cause remains unknown. Alcohol, tobacco, chronic local trauma, and Candida albicans are important predisposing factors.
Clinical features - Three clinical varieties are recognized: homogenous (common), speckled (less common), and verrucous (rare). Speckled and verrucous leukoplakia have a greater risk for malignant transformation than the homogenous type. The average percentage of malignant transformation for leukoplakia varies between 4% and 6%.
Laboratory tests - biopsy and histopathological examination
Treatment - Elimination of predisposing factors, systemic retinoid compounds. Surgical excision in the treatment of choice

Hairy Leukoplakia
Hairy leukoplakia is one of the most common and characteristic lesions of HIV infection. Rarely, it can also appear in immunosupressed patients after organ transplantation.
Cause - The Epstein-Barr virus seems to play a role in its pathogenicity.
Clinical Features - Hairy leukoplakia presents as a white asymptomatic, often elevated and unremovable patch. The lesion is almost always found bilaterally on

the sides (lateral margins) of the tongue, and may spread to the top surfaces (dorsum) and bottom surfaces (ventral) of the tongue. Usually the surface of the lesion is corrugated with a vertical orientation. However, smooth and flat lesions may be seen. The lesion is not precancerous.
Treatment - Not required; however, in some cases, acyclovir may be used.

Lichen Planus
Lichen Planus is a relatively common chronic inflammatory condition of the oral mucosa and skin.
Cause - The cause is not well-known. It is believed that there is a T-cell mediated auto-immune process involved.
Clinical features - White papules that usually coalesce, forming a network of lines (Whickman's striae), are the characteristic oral lesions of the disease. Six forms of the disease are recognized in the oral mucosa: reticular or erosive (common), atrophic or hypertrophic (less common), bullous (rare). Middle-age individuals are more commonly affected (Men to women ratio 2:3). The inside of the cheeks, the tongue, and gums are the areas it tends to localize in. Skin lesions typically appear as polygonal purple papules. The prognosis is usually very good. Malignant transformation remains controversial.
Laboratory Tests - Biopsy and histopathological examination is often very helpful. Direct immunofluorecence may also be used.
Treatment - No treatment is needed in asymptomatic lesions. Topical steroids (ointment in Orabase, intralesional injection) may also be helpful. Systemic steroids in low doses can be used in severe and extensive cases. The topical use of antiseptic mouthwashes should be avoided.

Linea Alba
Linea alba is a relatively common alteration of the buccal mucosa (the inside of the cheeks).
Cause - Pressure; sucking from the cheek surface of the teeth.
Clinical features - It presents as an asymptomatic, bilateral, linear elevation with a slightly whitish color at the level of the occlusal line of the teeth. Diagnosis is based on clinical evaluation alone.
Treatment - No treatment is required.

Nicotine Stomatitis
Smoker's palate or nicotine stomatitis is a common tobacco related type of keratosis that exclusively occurs on the hard palate and is typically associated with pipe and cigar smoking.
Cause - It's the temperature, not the chemicals in the smoke that is responsible.
Clinical features - Clinically, the palatal mucosa responds initially with redness. Later it becomes wrinkled and takes on a diffuse whitish-gray color with numerous micronodules of inflamed and dilated salivary gland ducts. These lesions are not premalignant, in contrast to the "reverse smoker's palate," which is associated with reverse smoking.

Laboratory tests - Usually none are required.
Treatment - Smoking cessation

Chemical Burn
This is an injury to the oral mucosa caused by topical application of caustic agents.
Cause - Common causative agents include - hydrogen peroxide, aspirin and alcohol.
Clinical features - Clinically, the affected area is covered by a whitish membrane (due to necrosis/ cell death). The dead mucosa can be easily scrapped off, leaving a red bleeding surface. The lesions are painful. Diagnosis should be made on the basis of clinical features and history.
Treatment - purely symptomatic.

Candidiasis
Candidiasis is the most common oral fungal infection.
Cause - It is usually caused by Candida albicans, and less frequently by other fungal species. Predisposing factors include poor hygiene, xerostomia (dry mouth), dentures, antibiotic mouthwashes, broad-spectrum antibiotics, steroids, radiation, HIV infection, iron-deficiency anemia, and endocrine disorders.
Treatment - Topical antifungal agents (nystatin nd amphoteracin B), systemic azoles.

Chronic Biting
Mild chronic biting of the oral mucosa is relatively common in nervous individuals. These patients consciously bite the inside surface of their cheeks, lips and tongue and detach the superficial epithelial (skin) layers.
Clinical features - The lesions are characterized by a diffuse irregular white area of small furrows. Rarely, erosion and bruising may be seen. Diagnosis is made clinically.
Treatment - Encouragement to stop the habit.

Geographic Tongue
Geographic tongue is a relatively common benign condition, particularly affecting the tongue and rarely other oral mucosal sites.
Cause - Unknown.
Clinical Features - Clinically, the condition is characterized by multiple well demarcated, red, depapillated patches, typically surrounded by a slightly elevated whitish border and usually restricted to the dorsum (top) of the tongue. Usually the lesions persist for a short time in one area, then disappear completely and reappear in another area. The condition is usually asymptomatic and often coexists with fissured tongue. The diagnosis is made clinically.
Treatment - patient reassurance.

Hairy Tongue
Hairy tongue is a relatively common disorder that is due to marked accumulation of keratin on the filliform papillae of the tongue, resulting in a hair-like pattern.

Cause - Unknown. Predisposing factors include: poor oral hygiene, oxidizing mouthwashes, antibiotics, excessive smoking, emotional stress, radiation therapy, bacterial and fungal (Candida) infections.
Treatment - Elimination of predisposing factors. Tongue brushing and use of keratolytic agents.

Furred Tongue
Furred tongue is a relatively uncommon condition, usually appearing during febrile illness.
Cause - Unknown. Predisposing factors are febrile painful oral lesions, poor oral hygiene, dehydration, and a soft diet.
Clinical features - Clinically, it appears as a white or whitish-yellow thick coating on the surface of the tongue. The lesion is due to the lengthening of the filiform papillae (up to 3 to 4 mm) and accumulation of debris and bacteria. Usually, the condition appears and disappears within a short period of time. Diagnosis is made clinically.
Treatment - Therapy of the underlying illness and improvement of oral hygiene.

Material Alba
Material alba results from the accumulation of food debris, dead epithelial cells, and bacteria. It is common at the dentogingival margin.
Cause - poor oral hygiene
Clinical features - It presents as a soft whitish plaque that is easily detached after slight pressure.

Treatment - good oral hygiene

Fordyce's Granules
Fordyce's granules are ectopic sebacceous glands of the oral mucosa.
Cause - normal anatomical variation.
Clinical features - They present as multiple, asymptomatic, slightly raised whitish-yellow spots. The vermillion border of the upper lip and the insides of the cheeks are the common sites of predilection. They occur in about 80% of adults of both sexes.
Treatment - None required.

Leukoedema
Leukoedema is a normal anatomic variation.
Cause - It is due to increased thickness of the epithelium and intracellular edema (swelling) of the prickle-cell layer.
Clinical Features - Clinically, it is characterized by a grayish-white, opalescent pattern of the mucosa and a slightly wrinkling surface. It usually occurs bilaterally on the inside of the cheeks and rarely on the tongue and lips.
Treatment - None required.

White Spongy Nevus

White spongy nevus is a relatively rare inherited trait.

Clinical features - It presents as symmetrical white lesions with multiple furrows and a spongy texture. The lesions may appear at birth, or more commonly at early childhood. The insides of the cheeks and the surfaces under the tongue are the sites of predilection.

Treatment - None required.

Papilloma

Papilloma appears as a exophytic, painless, usually pedunculated growth. Characteristically the tumor has a white or normal color, with numerous finger-like projections that form a cauliflower pattern. Papilloma is usually solitary with an average size of 0.5 - 1cm.

Verrucous Carcinoma

Verrucous carcinoma is a low grade variant of squamous cell carcinoma. Presumably, human papillomavirus is involved in the pathogenesis.

Clinical Features - Clinically, it presents as a white mass with a pebbly surface. The size varies from 1cm in the early stages to very extensive lesions. The cheek, palate and gums are the most common sites of involvement. The condition mainly develops in smokers over the age of 60.

Laboratory tests - biopsy.

Treatment - Surgical excision.

Squamous Cell Carcinoma

Squamous cell carcinoma has a wide spectrum of clinical features. In about 5% to 8% of cases, it appears in the early stages as a white, asymetric plaque similar to leukoplakia. Biopsy and histopathological examination are important for the diagnosis in these cases.

TMJ Review

The temporomandibular joint, or TMJ, is the articulation between the condyle of the mandible and the squamous portion of the temporal bone.

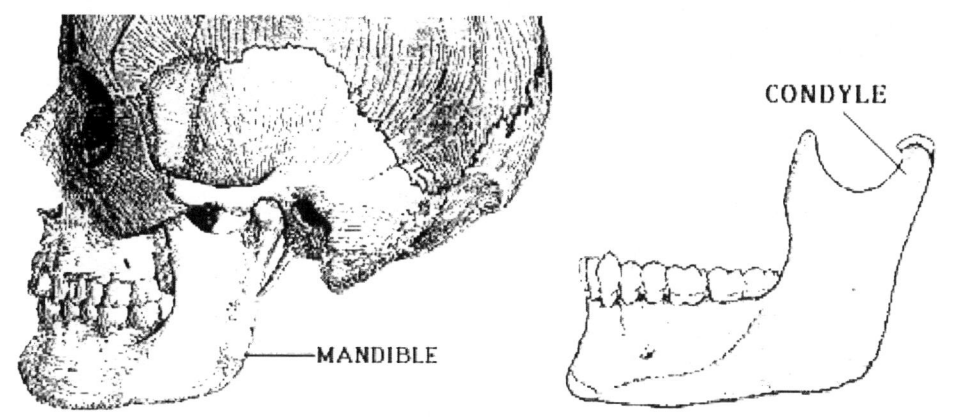

The condyle is elliptically shaped with its long axis oriented mediolaterally.

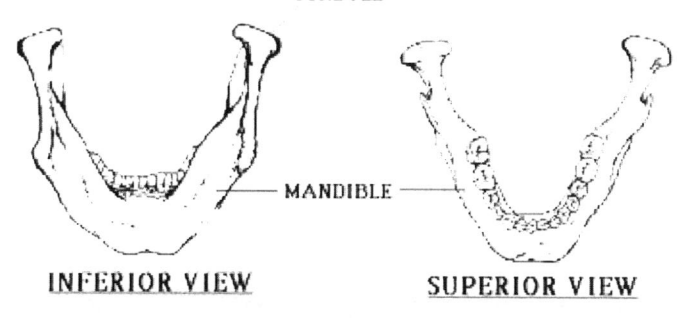

The articular surface of the temporal bone is composed of the concave articular fossa and the convex articular eminence.

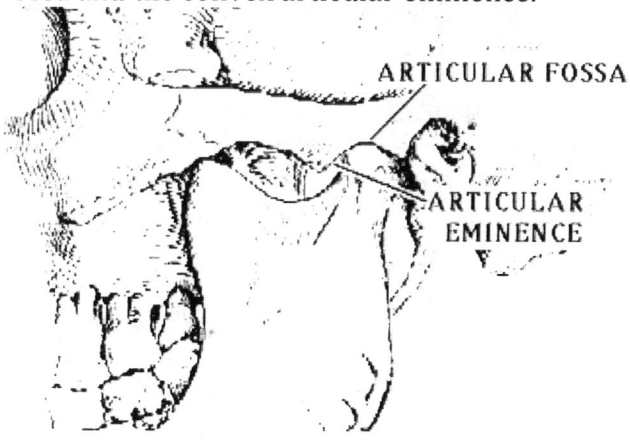

The meniscus is a fibrous, saddle shaped structure that separates the condyle and the temporal bone. The meniscus varies in thickness: the thinner, central intermediate zone separates thicker portions called the anterior band and the posterior band. Posteriorly, the meniscus is contiguous with the posterior attachment tissues called the bilaminar zone. The bilaminar zone is a vascular, innervated tissue that plays an important role in allowing the condyle to move foreward. The meniscus and its attachments divide the joint into superior and inferior spaces. The superior joint space is bounded above by the articular fossa and the articular eminence. The inferior joint space is bounded below by the condyle. Both joint spaces have small capacities, generally 1cc or less.

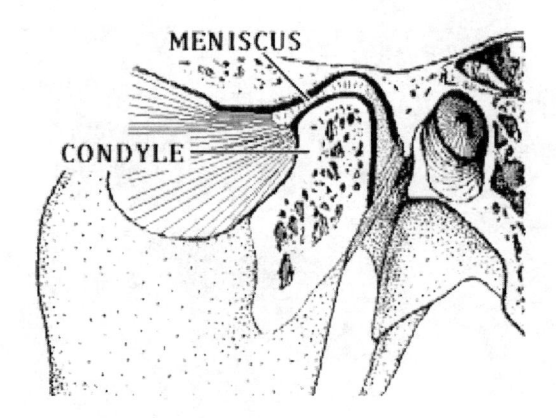

Normal TMJ Function

When the mouth opens, two distinct motions occur at the joint. The first motion is rotation around a horizontal axis through the condylar heads. The second motion is translation. The condyle and meniscus move together anteriorly beneath the articular eminence. In the closed mouth position, the thick posterior band of the meniscus lies immediately above the condyle. As the condyle translates forward, the thinner intermediate zone of the meniscus becomes the articulating surface between the condyle and the articular eminence. When the mouth is fully open, the condyle may lie beneath the anterior band of the meniscus.

TMJ Dysfunction

Internal derangement of the TMJ is present when the posterior band of the meniscus is anteriorly displaced in front of the condyle. As the meniscus translates anteriorly, the posterior band remains in front of the condyle and the bilaminar zone becomes abnormally stretched and attenuated. Often the displaced posterior band will return to its normal position when the condyle reaches a certain point. This is termed anterior displacement with reduction.

When the meniscus reduces the patient often feels a pop or click in the joint. In some patients the meniscus remains anteriorly displaced at full mouth opening. This is termed anterior displacement without reduction. Patients with anterior displacement without reduction often cannot fully open their mouths'. Sometimes there is a tear or perforation of the meniscus. Grinding noises in the joint are often present.

Major Functions of Cells Mediating Immune Responses

Neutrophils-phagocytosis, release chemicals involved in inflammation (vasodilators, chemotaxins)

Basophils-have functions in blood similar to those of mast cells in tissues

Eosinophils- destroy multicellular parasites, participate in immediate hypersensitivity reactions

Monocytes- have functions in blood similar to those of macrophages in tissues, enter tissues and are transformed into macrophages

B cells-initiate antibody-mediated immune responses by binding specific antigens to their plasma-membrane receptors, which are immunoglobulins. During activation are transformed into plasma cells, which secrete antibodies, present antigen to helper T cells.

Cytotoxic T cells- bind to antigens on plasma membrane of target cells (virus-infected cells, cancer cells and tissue transplants) and directly destroy the cells

Helper T cells-secrete cytokines that help to activate B cells, cytotoxic T cells, NK cells, and macrophages

NK cells-bind directly and nonspecifically to virus-infected cells and cancer cells and kill them, function as killer cells in antibody-dependent cellular cytotoxicity

Plasma cells-secrete antibodies

Macrophages and macrophage-like cells-Phagocytosis and intracellular killing, extracellular killing via secretion of toxic chemicals, process and present antigens to helper T-cells, secrete cytokines involved in inflammation, activation and differentiation of helper T cells, and systemic responses to infection or injury (the acute phase response)

Mast cells- release histamine and other chemicals involved in inflammation

Anatomic Sciences

Axial Skeleton

The axial skeleton consists of 80 bones forming the trunk (spine and thorax) and skull.

Vertebral Column: The main trunk of the body is supported by the spine, or vertebral column, which is composed of 26 bones, some of which are formed by the fusion of a few bones. The vertebral column from superior to inferior consists of 7 cervical (neck), 12 thoracic and 5 lumbar vertebrae, as well as a sacrum, formed by fusion of 5 sacral vertebrae, and a coccyx, formed by fusion of 4 coccygeal vertebrae.

Ribs and Sternum: The axial skeleton also contains 12 pairs of *ribs* attached posteriorly to the thoracic vertebrae and anteriorly either directly or via cartilage to the *sternum* (breastbone). The ribs and sternum form the *thoracic cage*, which protects the heart and lungs. Seven pairs of ribs articulate with the sternum (*fixed ribs*) directly, and three do so via cartilage; the two most inferior pairs do not attach anteriorly and are referred to as *floating ribs*.

Skull: The skull consists of 22 bones fused together to form a rigid structure which houses and protects organs such as the brain, auditory apparatus and eyes. The bones of the skull form the *face* and *cranium* (brain case) and consist of 6 single bones (*occipital, frontal, ethmoid, sphenoid, vomer* and *mandible*) and 8 paired bones (*parietal, temporal, maxillary, palatine, zygomatic, lacrimal, inferior concha* and *nasal*). The *lower jaw* or *mandible* is the only movable bone of the skull (head); it articulates with the temporal bones.

Other Parts: Other bones considered part of the axial skeleton are the *middle ear bones* (*ossicles*) and the small U-shaped *hyoid bone* that is suspended in a portion of the neck by muscles and ligaments.

Appendicular Skeleton

The *appendicular skeleton* forms the major internal support of the appendages—the *upper* and *lower extremities* (limbs).

Pectoral Girdle and Upper Extremities: The arms are attached to and suspended from the axial skeleton via the *shoulder* (*pectoral*) *girdle*. The latter is composed of two *clavicles* (*collarbones)* and two *scapulae* (*shoulder blades*). The clavicles articulate with the sternum; the two *sternoclavicular joints* are the only sites of articulation between the trunk and upper extremity.

Each upper limb from distal to proximal (closest to the body) consists of hand, wrist, forearm and arm (upper arm). The *hand* consists of 5 *digits* (fingers) and 5 *metacarpal* bones. Each digit is composed of three bones called *phalanges*, except the thumb which has only two bones.

Pelvic Girdle and Lower Extremities: The lower *extremities*, or legs, are attached to the axial skeleton via the *pelvic* or *hip girdle*. Each of the two coxal, or *hip bones* comprising the pelvic girdle is formed by the fusion of three bones—*illium, pubis, and ischium.* The coxal bones attach the lower limbs to the trunk by articulating with the sacrum.

THE HUMAN SKELETAL SYSTEM	
Part of the Skeleton	**Number of Bones**
Axial Skeleton	**80**
Skull	22
Ossicles (malleus, incus and stapes)	6
Vertebral column	26
Ribs	24
Sternum	1
Hyoid	1
Appendicular Skeleton	**126**
Upper extremities	64
Lower extremities	62

Characteristics of Bone

Bone is a specialized type of connective tissue consisting of cells (*osteocytes*) embedded in a calcified matrix which gives bone its characteristic hard and rigid nature. Bones are encased by a *periosteum*, a connective tissue sheath. All bone has a central marrow cavity. *Bone marrow* fills the marrow cavity or smaller marrow spaces, depending on the type of bone.

Types of Bone: There are two types of bone in the skeleton: *compact bone* and *spongy* (cancellous) bone.

Compact Bone. Compact bone lies within the periosteum, forms the outer region of bones, and appears dense due to its compact organization. The living osteocytes and calcified matrix are arranged in layers, or *lamellae*. Lamellae may be circularly arranged surrounding a central canal, the *Haversian canal*, which contains small blood vessels.

Spongy Bone. Spongy bone consists of *bars, spicules* or *trabeculae*, which forms a lattice meshwork. Spongy bone is found at the ends of long bones and the inner layer of flat, irregular and short bones. The trabeculae consist of osteocytes embedded in calcified matrix, which in definitive bone has a lamellar nature. The spaces between the trabeculae contain bone marrow.

Bone Cells: The cells of bone are osteocytes, osteoblasts, and osteoclasts. *Osteocytes* are found singly in *lacunae* (spaces) within the calcified matrix and communicate with each other via small canals in the bone known as *canaliculi*. The latter contain osteocyte cell processes. The osteocytes in compact and spongy bone are similar in structure and function.

Osteoblasts are cells which form bone matrix, surrounding themselves with it, and thus are transformed into osteocytes. They arise from undifferentiated cells, such as mesenchymal cells. They are cuboidal cells which line the trabeculae of immature or developing spongy bone.

Osteoclasts are cells found during bone development and remodeling. They are multinucleated cells lying in cavities, *Howship's lacunae*, on the surface of the bone tissue being resorbed. Osteoclasts remove the existing calcified matrix releasing the inorganic or organic components.

Bone Matrix: *Matrix* of compact and spongy bone consists of collagenous fibers and ground substance which constitute the organic component of bone. Matrix also consists of inorganic material which is about 65% of the dry weight of bone. Approximately 85% of the inorganic component consists of calcium phosphate in a crystalline form (hydroxyapatite crystals). Glycoproteins are the main components of the ground substance.

MAJOR TYPES OF HUMAN BONES

Type of Bone	Characteristics	Examples
Long bones	Width less than length	Humerus, radius, ulna, femur, tibia
Short bones	Length and width close to equal in size	Carpal and tarsal bones
Flat bones	Thin flat shape	Scapulae, ribs, sternum, bones of cranium (occipital, frontal, parietal)
Irregular bones	Multifaceted shape	Vertebrae, sphenoid, ethmoid

| Sesamoid | Small bones located in tendons of muscles | --------- |

Joints

The bones of the skeoeton articulate with each other at *joints*, which are variable in structure and function. Some joints are immovable, such as the *sutures* between the bones of the cranium. Others are *slightly movable joints*; examples are the *intervertebral joints* and the *pubic symphysis* (joint between the two pubic bones of the coxal bones).

TYPES OF JOINTS

Joint Type	Characteristic	Example
Ball and socket	Permits all types of movement (abduction, adduction, flexion, extension, circumduction); it is considered a universal joint.	Hips and shoulder joints
Hinge (ginglymus)	Permits motion in one plane only	Elbow and knee, interphalangeal joints
Rotating or pivot	Rotation is only motion permitted	Radius and ulna, atlas and axis (first and second cervical vertebrae)
Plane or gliding	Permits sliding motion	Between tarsal bones and carpal bones
Condylar (condyloid)	Permits motion in two planes which are at right angles to each other (rotation is not possible)	Metacarop-phalangeal joints, temporomandibular

Adjacent bones at a joint are connected by fibrous connective tissue bands known as *ligaments*. They are strong bands which support the joint and may also act to limit the degree of motion occurring at a joint.

Four Basic Tissues

1. **Muscle Tissue:** Muscle tissue is contractile in nature and functions to move the skeletal system and body viscera.

TYPES OF MUSCLE

Type	Characteristics	Location
Skeletal	Striated, voluntary	Skeletal muscles of the body
Smooth	Non-striated, involuntary	Walls of digestive tract and blood vessels, uterus, urinary bladder
Cardiac	Striated, involuntary	heart

2. **Nervous Tissue:** Nervous tissue is composed of cells (*neurons*) that respond to external and internal stimuli and have the capability to transmit a message (*impulse*) from one area of the body to another. This tissue thus induces a response of distant muscles or glands, as well as regulating body processes such as respiration, circulation, and digestion.

3. **Epithelial Tissue:** Epithelial tissue covers the external surfaces of the body and lines the internal tubes and cavities. It also forms the glands of the body. Characteristics of epithelial tissue (epithelium) are that it
    (1) has compactly aggregated cells;
    (2) has limited intercellular spaces and substance;
    (3) is avascular (no blood vessels);
    (4) lies on a connective tissue layer—the basal lamina;
    (5) has cells that form sheets and are polarized;
    (6) is derived from all three germ layers.

TYPES OF EPITHELIUM

Classification	Location(s)	Function(s)
Simple squamous epithelium	Endothelium of blood and lymphatic vessels; Bowman's capsule and thin loop of Henle in kidney; mesothelium lining pericardial, peritoneal and pleural body cavities; lung alveoli;	Lubrication of body cavities (permits free movement of organs); pinocytotic transports across cells

	smallest excretory ducts of glands	
Stratified squamous keratinized epithelium	Epidermis of skin	Prevents loss of water and protection
Stratified squamous nonkeratinized epithelium (moist)	Mucosa of oral cavity, esophagus, anal canal; vagina; cornea of eye and part of conjunctiva	Secretion; protection; prevents loss of water
Simple cuboidal epithelium	Kidney tubules; choroids plexus; thyroid gland; rete testis; surface of ovary	Secretion; absorption; lines surface
Stratified cuboidal epithelium	Ducts of sweat glands; developing follicles of ovary	Secretion; protection
Simple columnar epithelium	Cells lining lumen of digestive tract (stomach to rectum); gall bladder; many glands (secretory units and ducts); uterus; uterine tube (ciliated)	Secretion; absorption; protection; lubrication
Pseudostratified columnar epithelium	Lines lumen of respiratory tract (nasal cavity, trachea and bronchi) (ciliated); ducts of epididymis (stereocilia); ductus deferens; male urethra	Secretion; protection; facilitates transport of substances on surface of cells
Stratified columnar epithelium	Male urethra; conjunctiva	Protection
Transitional epithelium	Urinary tract (renal calyces and pelvis, ureter and urinary bladder)	Protection

Epithelial cells may also have specializations at the cell surface. For example,

Microvilli—fingerlike projections of plasma membranes.

Cilia—motile organelles extending into the luman consisting of specifically arranged microtubules.
Flagella—similar to cilia. Primary examples are human spermatozoa.
Stereocilia—are actually very elongated Microvilli.

4. **Connective Tissue:** Connective tissue is the packing and supporting material of the body tissues and organs. It develops from mesoderm (mesenchyme). All connective tissues consist of three distinct components: ground substance, cells and fibers.

    a) *Ground substance.* Ground substance is located between the cells and fibers, both of which are embedded in it. It forms an amorphous intercellar material. In the fresh state, it appears as a transparent and homogenous gel. It acts as a route for the passage of nutrients and wastes to and from the cells within or adjacent to the connective tissue.

    b) *Fibers.* The fiber components of connective tissue add support and strength. Three types of fibers are present: *collagenous, elastic* and *reticular*.

Integumentary (Skin) System

The skin and the specialized organs derived from the skin (hair, nails and glands) form the integumentary system.

Functions: The skin functions by surfacing the body and thus protecting it from dehydration as well as from damage by the elements in the external environment. The skin also helps maintain normal body activities.

Structure: Skin consists of the *epidermis* and *dermis* (*corium*). Deep to the dermis and therefore, the skin, is the *hypodermis*, which is also known as the *subcutaneous* or superficial connective tissue of the body.

Epidermis: The epidermis is derived from the ectoderm and is composed of a keratinized stratified squamous epithelium. *Thick skin* denotes skin with a thicker epidermis which contains more cell layers when compared to *thin skin*. The epidermis ranges in thickness from 0.07 millimeter to 1.4 millimeters. The epidermis consists of specific cell layers:

1. stratum basale or germinativum
2. stratum spinosum
3. stratum granulosum
4. stratum lucidum
5. stratum corneum

Glands

Glands are specialized organs derived from skin. There are two basic types: sebaceous and sweat.

Sebaceous Glands: Sebaceous glands are *simple branched alveolar* (*acinar*) *glands* with a *holocrine* mode of secretion.

Sweat Glands: Sweat is a watery fluid containing ammonia, urea, uric acid and sodium chloride. There are two types of sweat glands: eccrine and apocrine.

Eccrine Sweat Glands: The *eccrine sweat glands* are simple, coiled tubular glands with a merocrine mode of secretion.

Apocrine Sweat Glands: the *apocrine sweat glands* are very large glands which are thought to have a merocrine mode of secretion.

Hair

Hairs are long, filamentous keratinized structures derived from the epidermis of skin.

Structure: A hair consists of a *shaft* and a *root*.

Hair Follicles: The *hair follicle* consists of two sheathes, the *epithelial root sheath* and the *connective tissue root sheath*.

Hair Growth: Growth of a hair depends on the viability of the epidermal cells of the hair matrix which lie adjacent to the dermal papilla in the hair bulb. The matrix cells abutting the dermal papilla proliferate and give rise to cells which move upward to become part of the specific layers of the hair root and the inner epithelial root sheath.

Hair Musculature: Hairs are oriented at a slight angle to the skin surface and are associated with *arrector pili muscles*. These smooth muscle bundles extend from the dermal root sheath to a dermal papilla. Contraction results in the standing up of the hairs and raising of the skin surrounding the hair.

Nails

Nails are translucent plates of keratinized epithelial cells on the dorsal surface of distal phalanges of fingers and toes.

Muscles of Mastication

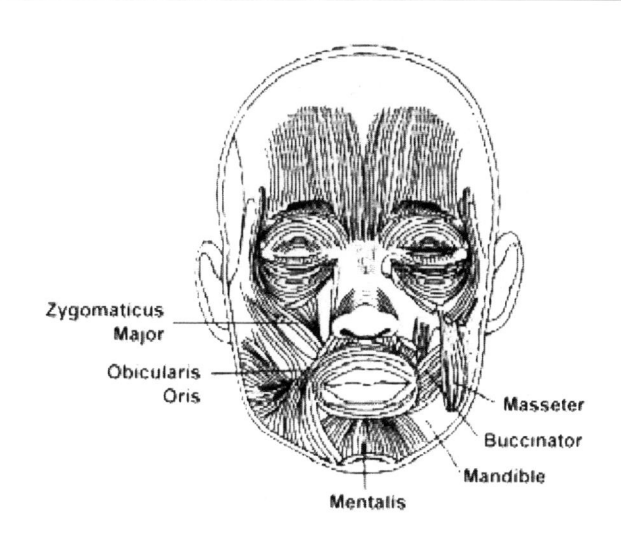

Muscle	Origin	Insertion	Function
Masseter	Zygomatic arch	Mandible (external surface)	Closes the jaw
Temporalis	Temporal bone	Coronoid Process at the anterior border of the ramus	Closes the jaw
Medial Ptyergoid	Sphenoid, palatine and maxillary bones	Medial surface of the ramus	Closes the jaw
Lateral Ptyergoid	Sphenoid bones	Anterior surface iof the mandibular condyle	Opens the jaw, grinding action side to side, protrusion

Muscles of Expression

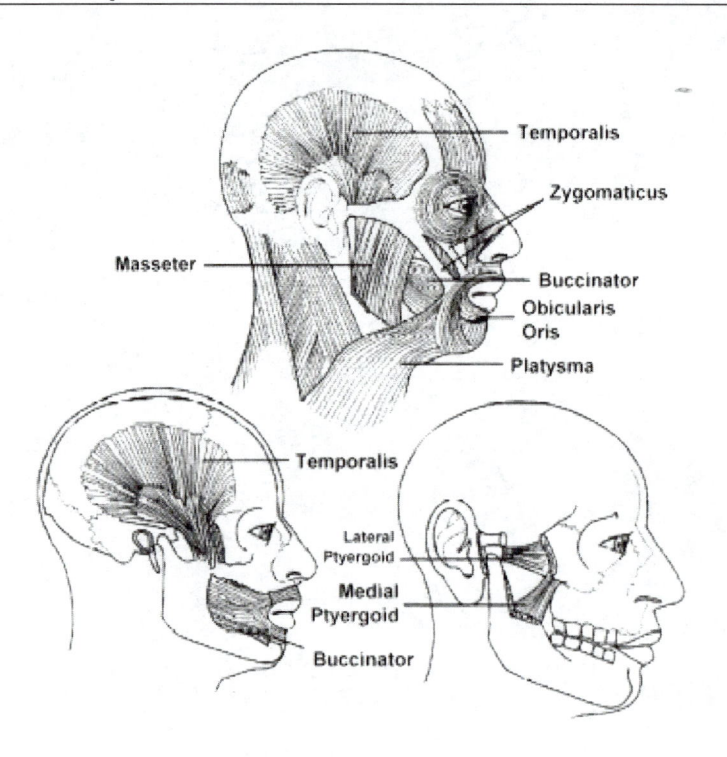

Muscle	Origin	Insertion	Function
Buccinator	Alveolar process of mand. and max	Obicularis oris at the corner of the mouth	Holds food in contact with the teeth when chewing
Obicularis oris	No attachment to bone	Corners of the mouth	Closes the lips
Mentalis	Mandible	skin of the chin	Protrudes the lower lip
Zygomaticus major	Zygomatic bone	Obicularis oris	Raises the corner of the mouth when smiling

Neurology Review

Brain

Frontal lobe-controls emotions, judgments, controls motor aspects of speech, primary motor cortex for voluntary muscle activation

Parietal lobe-receives fibers with sensory information about touch, proprioception, temperature, and pain from the other side of the body

Temporal lobe-responsible for auditory information, and language comprehension

Occipital lobe- center for visual information
Cerebellum- coordination of muscle function
Brainstem - (midbrain, pons, and medulla)-respiratory and cardiac center, nerve pathways to the brain

間腦 *Diencephalon – (thalamus, subthalamus, and hypothalamus)*
　　　　　視丘　　　　　　　　　　下視丘

Thalamus – Integrate and relay sensory information from the face, retina, cochlea, and taste receptors. (Interprets sensation of touch, pain and temperature).
Hypothalamus
1. Controls the autonomic nervous system and the neuroendocrine systems.
2. Maintains body homeostasis
3. Helps regulate body temperature
4. Helps regulate appetite control
5. Thirst Center
6. Sleeping Cycle
7. Control of Hormone secretion

Autonomic Nervous System
Sympathetic (Fight or Flight):
1. Dilated pupils
2. Elevates heart rate and respiratory rate
3. Sweating
4. Epinephrine and norepinephrine secreted
5. Increased blood pressure
6. Constriction of skin and abdominal arterioles

Parasympathetic:
1. Constricted pupils
2. Lowers heart rate and respiratory rate
3. Increased peristalsis
4. Acetylcholine secreted
5. Decreases blood pressure
6. Relaxation of skin and abdominal arterioles

Cranial Nerves
I-Olfactory-Smell
II-Optic-Vision acuity
III-Oculomotor – Eye function
IV-Trochlear – Eye function
V-Trigeminal – Sensory of the face, chewing
VI-Abducens – Eye function
VII-Facial – Facial expression, wrinkle forehead, taste anterior tongue

VIII-Vestibulocochlear – Auditory acuity, balance and postural responses
IX-Glossopharyngeal – taste on posterior 33% of the scale
X-Vagus – Cardiac, respiratory reflexes
XI-Spinal Accessory - Strength of trapezius and Sternocleidomastoid muscles
XII-Hypoglossal – Motor function of the tongue

Decorticate vs. Decerebrate Rigidity
Decorticate posturing-Upper limbs in flexion and the lower limbs in extension
Decerebrate posturing- Increased tone with all limbs in a position of extension

Key Terms
- Apraxia-Inability to perform purposeful movements
- Agnosia-Inability to recognize familiar objects by the various senses
- Spasticity-increased tone, hyperactive reflexes, clonus,+Babinski
- Ataxia-general term used to describe uncoordinated movement; may influence gait, posture, and patterns of movements
- Chorea-involuntary, rapid, irregular, jerky movements, clinical feature of Huntington disease
- Flaccidity-absent tone
- Hypotonia-decreased tone
- Expressive Aphasia- inability to speak or difficulty speaking
- Receptive Aphasia-inability to understand verbal speech, inability to receive information

CVA, Stroke
1. Anterior cerebral stroke: lower extremity more involved than upper extremity, contralateral hemiparesis and sensory deficits
2. Posterior cerebral stroke: contralateral sensory loss, transient contralateral hemiparesis
3. Middle cerebral artery stroke: upper extremity more involved than the lower extremity, contralateral sensory loss

Risk Factors
1. Diabetes
2. Atherosclerosis
3. Hypertension
4. Cardiac disease
5. Transient ischemic attacks

Aneurysm Precautions
1. Avoid rectal temperatures
2. Limit visitors
3. Avoid Valsalva's maneuver
4. Head of bed should be between 30-45 degrees

Valsalva's maneuver – occurs when attempting to forcibly exhale with the glottis, mouth and nose closed. It causes an increase in intrathoracic pressure with an accompanying collapse of the vein of the chest wall. The following may result:
1. Slowing of the pulse
2. Decreased return of blood to the heart
3. Increased intrathoracic pressure

Elevated Intracranial Pressure
In most cases you should do the following:
1. Maintain proper fluid volumes
2. Set-up quiet environment for minimal sensory stimulation
3. Elevate HOB (head of bed) to approximately 30 degrees
4. Limit suctioning performed

Horner's Syndrome- Sympathetic innervation to the face is interrupted by a lesion in the brain stem resulting in pupillary constriction, dry and red face with no sweat, ptosis-Mueller's muscle, problem located in sympathetic ascending fibers

Autonomic Dysreflexia- caused by a lesion in the high thoracic or cervical cord. Severe hypertension, sweating and headaches noted. May occur with a blockage in a urine catheter
Signs/Symptoms
1. Bradycardia
2. Headache
3. Increased parasympathetic activity
4. Excessive perspiration
5. Excessive sympathetic response
6. Elevated blood pressure
7. Stimulation of baroreceptors in aortic arch and caroticd sinus

*Parkinson's Disease-*a degenerative disease with primary involvement of the basal ganglia; characterized by the following:
Signs/Symptoms
1. Bradykinesia
2. Resting tremor
3. Impaired postural reflexes
4. Rigidity
5. Loss of inhibitory dopamine
6. Mask like affect
7. Emotional lability

*Multiple Sclerosis-*progressive demyelinating disease of the central nervous system affecting mostly young adults
Cause unknown, most likely viral.
1. Fluctuating exacerbations

2. Demyelinating lesions limit neural transmission
3. Confirmed with lumbar puncture, elevated gamma globulin, CT/MRI, myelogram, EEG.
4. Mild to moderate impaired cognition common
5. Sensory Deficits
6. Bowel and Bladder Deficits
7. Spasticity common
8. Ataxic gait

Myasthenia gravis- neuromuscular disease characterized by fatigue of skeletal muscles and muscular weakness.

Signs/Symptoms
1. Progressive involvement
2. Decreased muscle membrane acetylcholine receptors
3. Severe weakness (proximal more than distal muscles)
4. Facial, ocular and bulbar weakness
5. Possible life-threatening respiratory muscle weakness
6. Probable use of anticholinesterase drugs for treatment

Guillain-Barre' Syndrome-polyneuropathy with progressive muscular weakness
Signs/Symptoms
1. Demyelination of peripheral and cranial nerves
2. Motor paralysis in an ascending pattern
3. 3% Mortality – respiratory failure
4. Autonomic dysfunction-arrhythmias, blood pressure changes, tachycardia

Amyotrophic lateral sclerosis (Lou Gehrig's disease) – degenerative disease affecting upper and lower motor neurons
Signs/Symptoms
1. Death typically in 2-5 yrs.
2. Spasticity, hyperreflexia
3. Dysarthria, Dysphagia
4. Autonomic Dysfunction in approximately 1/3 of patients
5. Cognition is normal

Post-polio Syndrome- slowly progressive muscle weakness that occurs in patients with a history of acute poliomyelitis, after a stable period
Sign/Symptoms
1. New Weakness
2. Pain/Myalgia
3. Abnormal fatigue

Seizures
Epilepsy-recurrent seizures due to excessive and sudden discharge of cerebral cortical neurons.
Tonic-clonic (Grand Mal) –Pt. confused and drowsy about the seizures, 2-5 min generally
Absence seizures (Petit Mal)- Brief, no convulsive contractions, may be up to 100X day
Simple Seizures- no loss of consciousness
Complex Seizures, brief loss of consciousness with psychomotor changes

**Key Point*- When a patient has a seizure during most interventions, do not use a tongue blade and allow free movement in a safe environment

Meningitis-inflammation of the meninges of the spinal cord and brain caused by bacteria.
The most common bacteria are the following: *Neisseria meningitidis, Diplococcus pneumoniae,* and *Haemophilus influenzae*
Signs/Symptoms
1. Brudzinski's sign
2. Kernig's sign
3. Stiff/Tight neck
4. Fever
5. Confused

Anterior Cord Syndrome – damage is mainly in anterior cord resulting in loss of motor function and pain and temperature with preservation of light touch, proprioception and position sense
Brown-Sequard Syndrome – hemisection of SC resulting in ipsilateral weakness and loss of position and vibration sense below the level of lesion

Upper Motor Neuron Lesion
    A. Disuse atrophy
    A. +Babinski
    B. Hypertonia (Spasticity)
    C. Weakness or paralysis of movement not individual muscles
    D. Hyperreflexia

Lower Motor Neuron Lesion
    A. True Atrophy
    B. Weakness of individual muscles
    C. Fibrillations
    D. Hyporeflexia

Reflex Arc

The typical pathway of a reflex may be outlined as follows: sensory receptor on dendrite of dorsal root ganglion cell --------→ ganglion cell ----------→ axon cell --------→ dorsal root --------→dorsal horn of spinal cord--------→ either directly to motor cell in ventral horn or via internuncial (association) neuron to ventral horn motor cell-------→ axon via ventral root ------→ spinal nerve-------→ effector organ (e.g., muscle).

Spinal Tracts

Ascending Pathways in the Posterior Funiculus
Fasciculus Gracicilis and Fasciculus Cuneatus - These pathways convey information on two point discrimination, vibration, and concious proprioception from nerves in the dorsal root ganglion to the ipsilateral nucleus gracilis and nucleus cuneatus, respectively, in the medulla oblongata where they synapse with secondary neurons. Fibers entering the tracts are added laterally and fibers originating in the lumbrosacral region are located most medially. The fasciculus gracilis is located medially, just adjacent to the posterior median septum, and contains axons arising from dorsal root ganglia T7 and below. The fasciculus cuneatus is located more laterally, between the fasciculus gracilis and the posterior horn of gray matter, and it contains axons from nerves in the dorsal root ganglia T6 and above. From the nucleii in the medulla, the axons of the secinary neurons cross to the contralateral side and progress to the posterior lateral nucleus of the thalamus where they synapse with neurons that project to the precentral gyrus.

Ascending Pathways in the Lateral Funiculus:
Lateral Spinothalamic - This tract carries sensations of pain and temperature from free nerve ending receptors throughout the body. Central processes of neurons, whose bodies are in the dorsal root ganglion, enter the cord at Lissauer's fasciculus, the white matter at the edge of the dorsal horn. From there they ascend the cord one or two spinal segments before entering the dorsal horn and synapsing with secondary neurons. These cross to the contralateral side through the white commisure and travel up the cord in the lateral spinothalamic tract located at the lateral aspect of the cord, just medial to the anterior spinocerebellar tract. As axons join the tract, they are added medially, so fibers relating to the lower body are in the lateral part of the tract. The secondary neurons ascend to several nuclei in the thalamus including the ventral posterior lateral nucleus (VPL) after giving off branches to the periaquiductal gray and reticular formation of the brain stem. These collaterals may play a role in pain transmission in the area.

Posterior Spinocerebellar and Cuneocerebellar - These tracts carry muscle position and movement information from muscle spindles and golgi tendon organs to the cerebellum. This tract never reaches the cerebrum and therefore the proprioception is unconscious. The posterior spinocerebellar tract is concerned with the lower half of the body, below C8, while the cueocerebellar tract is concerned with information above C8. From L3 to C8, primary neurons project into the posterior columns and synapse in a nucleus in the center gray matter called Clarke's column (which only exists in these segments). The secondary neurons send their axons laterally to the posterior spinocerebellar tract which ascends to the inferior cerebellar peduncle and into the cerebellum. Neurons entering the cord below the L3 level ascend in the posterior columns to L3, where they can go to Clarke's column. Primary neurons entering the cord higher than C8 enter the posterior column and synapse in the cuneate mucleus in the medulla. From there the secondary neurons continue rostrally as the cuneocerebellar tract, through the inferior penduncle and into the cerebellum.

Rostral Spinocerebellar and Anterior Spinocerebellar - These tracts carry postural information from muscle spindle and golgi tendon organs regarding an entire limb to the cerebellum. Primary neurons of the rostral spinocerebellar track have their cell bodies in the spinal root ganglia of lumbar and sacral nerves. They synapse at the base of the dorsal horn and the secondary neurons cross to the contralateral side of the cord and ascend the cord in the anterior spinocerebellar tract, passing through the superior penduncle into the cerebellum. The rostral spinocerebellar tract is the upper limb equivalent of the anterior spinothalamic tract. It has only been investigated in cats, so its pathway in humans is inferred. The primary neurons synapse at the base of the dorsal horn and the secondary neurons stay ipsilateral and ascend the cord in the rostral spinocerebellar tract, entering the cerebellum through either the inferior or superion penduncle.

Ascending Pathways of the Anterior Funiculus
Anterior Spinothalamic – This tract carries sensations of poorly localized crude touch, tickling, itching, and sex. It is continuous with the lateral spinothalamic and the separation between the two is not clearly defined. The primary neurons are receptors in the hairless skin of the body that have their cell bodies in the spinal ganglia and project into the posterior horn. There they synapse with secondary neurons that cross to the contralateral side of the cord and form the anterior spinothalamic tract. In the medulla this tract merges with the lateral spinothalamic tract and branches extensively to the reticular formation and lateral reticular nucleus. It ascends to the VPL nucleus and posterior region of the thalamus where the neurons synapse with tertiary neurons that project to the precentral gyrus of the cerebral cortex.

Descending Pathways
Lateral Corticispinal and Anterior Corticospinal – The corticospinal tract is the major descending pathway extending from the cerebral cortex and affecting both motor neurons and sensory interneurons in the spinal cord. The neurons arise from the primary motor cortex as well as the cortical areas of the parietal and temporal lobes. The axons descend from the cortex to become the internal capsule then continue caudally forming the pyramids in the medulla. At the junction between the medulla and spinal cord most (75 – 90%) of the fibers cross to the contralateral side forming the decussation of the pyramids. The crossed fibers continue their descent in the lateral funiculus as the lateral sorticospinal tract while the uncrossed fibers continue in the anterior funiculus as the anterior corticospinal tract. The anterior corticospinal tract usually does not extend past the thoracic segments and the fibers decussate at the cord segment where they terminate. About half of the fibers

synapse with interneurons at the base of the posterior horn to modify sensory input. The remaining half synapse with anterior horn motor neurons and adjacent interneurons. From there the anterior horn motor neurons terminate at neuromuscular junctions for voluntary muscle control.

Rubrospinal – This tract descends from the red nucleus in the midbrain, in the lateral funiculus of the cord, as far as the thoracic segments. It is important in controlling flexor tone in the limbs and serves as another connection of the cortex to the spinal cord through the inputs of the cerebral cortex and the cerebellum to the red nucleus. The tract runs closely with the lateral corticospinal tract. The fibers terminate on interneurons in the anterior gray horn which synapse with motor neurons.

Tectospinal – This tract begins at the superior colliculus of the midbrain, which is important for cisual-following and eye-centering reflexes and descends down under the periaquiductal gray, crossing the midline and forming the dorsal termental decussation. It continues caudally in the anterior funiculus as far as the cervical cord and the terminal fibers synapse with interneurons which synapse in turn with anterior horn motor neurons. The function of the tract is not well established, though it is thought to combine visial and auditory stimuli with postural reflex movements.

Reticulospinal Tracts – These two tracts arise from several layers in the brain stem reticular core and modify motor and sensory functions of the spinal cord. They can inhibit of fascilitale muscle activity and tone, influence respiration and circulation, and affect transmission on sensory impulses. The pontine reticulospinal tract originates at the pontine tegmentum and descends in the anterior funiculus, remaining uncrossed. The terminal fibers end on interneurons that project to both alpha motor neurons, affecting extrafusal muscle fibers, and gamma motor neurons, innervating intrafusal fibers of muscle spindles. The medullary reticulospinal tract arises from the medial 2/3 of the medulla and descends in the anterior funiculus, also remaining uncrossed. The terminal fibers go to interneurons that send their axons to both alpha and gamma motor neurons.

Vestibulospinal – This tract facilitales activity of extensor (antigravity) muscles providing basic posture. It arises from cells in the lateral vestibular nucleus in the medulla and descends ipsilaterally in the anterior funiculus. The vestibular nuclei all receive input from the vestibular organs of the inner ear and fromt he cerebellum. The tract gives off terminal fibers at each segment that synapse with interneurons , which project to anterior horn motor neurons.

Basal Ganglia Review

The basal ganglia form the major inputs to the ventral lateral nucleus of the thalamus, which in turn provides major inputs to area 6, comprised of the PMA and SMA, The basal ganglia is a collection of subcortical nuclei including the following:
caudate nucleus and putamen (called the striatum)
globus pallidus
subthalamus
substantia nigra

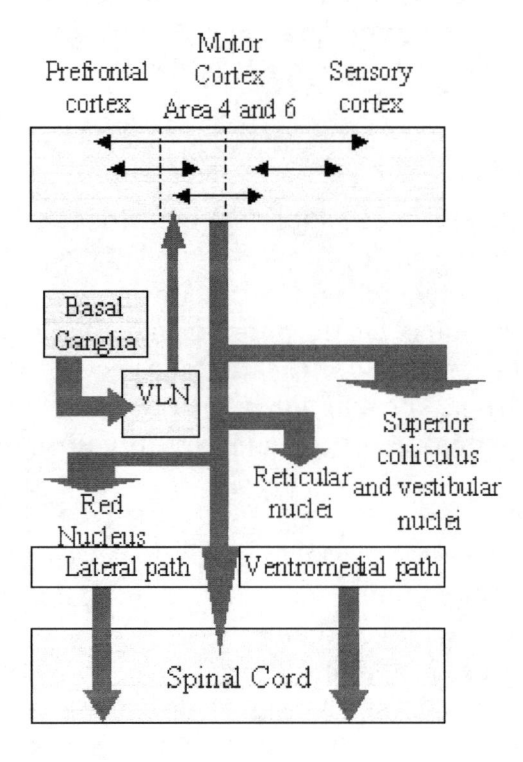

Respiratory/Cardiac Review

Normative Values for Infants/Adults

Term	Infant	Adult
HR	120bpm	60-100bpm
BP	75/50 mmHg	120/80 mmHg
RR	40	12-18
pH	7.26-7.41	7.35-7.45
Tidal Volume	20 ml	500 ml

COPD-Chronic Bronchitis/Emphysema-abnormal expiratory flow rates.

Chronic Bronchitis
Signs and Symptoms
1. Smoking History
2. Cor pulmonale
3. Decreased expiratory flow rates
4. Crackles and wheezes
5. Hypoxemia

Emphysema
Signs and Symptoms
1. Barralled chest
2. Dyspnea
3. Cyanosis
4. Clubbing
5. Accessory muscles of ventilation

Term	Obstructive Disease	Restrictive Disease
Total lung capacity	increases	decreases
Functional residual capacity	increases	decreases
Residual volume	increases	decreases
Vital capacity	decreases	decreases
PaCO2	increases	decreases

Tuberculosis-infectious respiratory process caused by tubercle bacilli.
Test-PPD-Purified Protein Derivative- Negative 0-4mm after 48 hours
Positive >10mm after 48 hrs.
Sputum + for *Mycobacterium tuberculosis* within 2-3 weeks of onset. Later (-) in the latent phase.
Drugs of choice in most cases Isoniazid and Rifampin.

Terminology

A. Orthopnea-difficulty breathing in positions other than upright sitting and standing
B. Orthostatic hypotension- decrease in blood pressure upon assuming an erect posture. This is normal, but may be excessive resulting in fainting.
C. Atelectasis-alveolar collapse involving part or all of the lung due to the complete absorption of gas or the inability of the alveoli to expand
D. Apnea- absence of respirations, usually temporary in duration
E. Bradycardia-Abnormally slow (low) pulse rate; below approximately 50 beats per minute.
F. Cor pulmonale-Right ventricular enlargement from a primary pulmonary cause
G. Cheyne-Strokes respiration-breathing pattern characterized by a gradual increase in rate and depth followed by a gradual decrease; periods of apnea occur between cycles.
H. Tachycardia-Abnormally rapid (high) pulse rate; over approximately 100 beats per minute.
I. Beta-adrenergic blocking agents (beta-blockers)-Propranolol, Metoprolol, nadolol, Atenolol, Timolol
J. Calcium channel blocking agent-Verapamil, Nifedipine, Diltiazem- A substance that inhibits the flow of calcium ions across membranes in smooth muscle. These drugs cause vasodilation and relieve angina pain and coronary artery spasm.
K. Ejection fraction-difference between left ventricular end diastolic volume and left ventricular end systolic volume.
L. Digitalis- a drug that strengthens the contraction of the heart muscle, slows the rate of contraction of the heart, and promotes the elimination of fluid from body tissues.
M. Antiarrhythmics-Lidocaine, Quinidine, Procainamide, Disopyramide, Phenytoin (Dilantin)- Agents used to treat cardiac arrhythmias.
N. Catecholamines-circulating compounds (epinephrine and norepinephrine) that are secreted by the sympathetic nervous system and the adrenal medulla; they act to increase cardiac rate, contractility, automaticity, and excitability.

Respiratory Conditions

The following respiratory information is not specifically on the NBDE exam. However, take the time to review the various conditions briefly so that you will be familiar with these terms in a hospital settting, a few may appear on the test.

ARDS- low oxygen levels caused by a build up of fluid in the lungs and inflammation of lung tissue.

Respiratory Acidosis- Build-up of Carbon Dioxide in the lungs that causes acid-base imbalances and the body becomes acidic.

Respiratory Alkalosis: CO2 levels are reduced and pH is high.

RSV (Respiratory synctial virus) - spread by contact, virus can survive for various time periods on different surfaces.

Apnea: no spontaneous breathing

Pneumonia: viruses the primary cause in young children, bacteria the primary cause in adults. Bacteria: Streptococcus pneumoniae, Mycoplasma pneumoniae *pneumoniae* (pneumococcus).

Pulmonary actinomycosis –bacteria infection of the lungs caused by (propionibacteria or actinomyces)

Alveolar proteinosis: A build-up of a phospholipid in the lungs were carbon dioxide and oxygen are transferred.

Pulmonary hypertension: elevated BP in the lung arteries

Pulmonary arteriovenous fistulas: a congenital defect were lung arteries and veins form improperly, and a fistula is formed creating poor oxygenation of blood.

Pulmonary aspergilloma: fungal infection of the lung cavities causing abscesses.

Pulmonary edema: most commonly caused by Heart Failure, but may be due to lung disorders.

Idiopathic pulmonary fibrosis: Thickening of lung tissue in the lower aspects of the lungs.

Pulmonary emboli: Blood clot of the pulmonary vessels or blockage due to fat droplets, tumors or parasites.

Tuberculosis- infection caused by *Mycobaterium tuberculosis*.

Causes:
Due to airborne exposure

Cytomegalovirus – can cause lung infections and is a herpes-type virus.

Viral pneumonia – inflammation of the lungs caused by viral infection.

Pneumothorax: a build-up of a gas in the pleural cavities.

Circulatory System

Functions

The circulatory system serves:

> (1) to conduct nutrients and oxygen to the tissues;
> (2) to remove waste materials by transporting nitrogenous compounds to the kidneys and carbon dioxide to the lungs;
> (3) to transport chemical messengers (hormones) to target organs and modulate and integrate the internal milieu of the body;
> (4) to transport agents which serve the body in allergic, immune, and infectious responses;
> (5) to initiate clotting and thereby prevent blood loss;
> (6) to maintain body temperature;
> (7) to produce, carry and contain blood;
> (8) to transfer body reserves, specifically mineral salts, to areas of need.

General Components and Structure

The circulatory system consists of the heart, blood vessels, blood and lymphatics. It is a network of tubular structures through which blood travels to and from all the parts of the body. In vertebrates this is a completely closed circuit system, as William Harvey (1628) once demonstrated. The heart is a modified, specialized, powerful pumping blood vessel. Arteries, eventually becoming arterioles, conduct blood to capillaries (essentially endothelial tubes), and venules, eventually becoming veins, return blood from the capillary bed to the heart.

Course of Circulation

Systemic Route:

a. *Arterial system.* Blood is delivered by the pulmonary veins (two from each lung) to the left atrium, passes through the bicuspid (mitral) valve into the left ventricle and then is pumped into the ascending aorta; backflow here is prevented by the aortic semilunar valves. The aortic arch toward the right side gives rise to the brachiocephalic (innominate) artery which divides into the right subclavian and right common carotid arteries. Next, arising from the arch is the common carotid artery, then the left subclavian artery.

The subclavians supply the upper limbs. As the subclavian arteries leave the axilla (armpit) and enter the arm (brachium), they are called brachial arteries. Below the elbow these main trunk lines divide into ulnar and radial arteries, which supply the forearm and eventually form a set of arterial arches in the hand which give rise to common and proper digital arteries. The descending (dorsal) aorta continues along the posterior aspect of the thorax giving rise to the segmental intercostals arteries. After passage "through" (behind) the diaphragm it is called the abdominal aorta.

At the pelvic rim the abdominal aorta divides into the right and left common iliac arteries. These divide into the internal iliacs, which supply the pelvic organs, and the external iliacs, which supply the lower limb.

b. *Venous system*. Veins are frequently multiple and variations are common. They return blood originating in the capillaries of peripheral and distal body parts to the heart.

Hepatic Portal System: Blood draining the alimentary tract (intestines), pancreas, spleen and gall bladder does not return directly to the systemic circulation, but is relayed by the hepatic portal system of veins to and through the liver. In the liver, absorbed foodstuffs and wastes are processed. After processing, the liver returns the blood via hepatic veins to the inferior vena cava and from there to the heart.

Pulmonary Circuit: Blood is oxygenated and depleted of metabolic products such as carbon dioxide in the lungs.

Lymphatic Drainage: A network of lymphatic capillaries permeates the body tissues. Lymph is a fluid similar in composition to blood plasma, and tissue fluids not reabsorbed into blood capillaries are transported via the lymphatic system eventually to join the venous system at the junction of the left internal jugular and subclavian veins.

The Heart

The heart is a highly specialized blood vessel which pumps 72 times per minute and propels about 4,000 gallons (about 15,000 liters) of blood daily to the tissues. It is composed of:
    Endocardium (lining coat; epithelium)
    Myocardium (middle coat; cardiac muscle)
    Epicardium (external coat or visceral layer of pericardium; epithelium and mostly connective tissue)
    Impulse conducting system

Cardiac Nerves: Modification of the intrinsic rhythmicity of the heart muscle is produced by cardiac nerves of the sympathetic and parasympathetic nervous system. Stimulation of the sympathetic system increases the rate and force of the heartbeat and dilates the coronary arteries. Stimulation of the parasympathetic (vagus nerve) reduces the rate and force of the heartbeat and constricts the coronary circulation. Visceral afferent (sensory) fibers from the heart end almost wholly in the first four segments of the thoracic spinal cord.

Cardiac Cycle: Alternating contraction and relaxation is repeated about 75 times per minute; the duration of one cycle is about 0.8 second. Three phases succeed one another during the cycle:
- a) atrial systole: 0.1 second,
- b) ventricular systole: 0.3 second,
- c) diastole: 0.4 second

The actual period of rest for each chamber is 0.7 second for the atria and 0.5 second for the ventricles, so in spite of its activity, the heart is at rest longer than at work.

Blood

Blood is composed of cells (corpuscles) and a liquid intercellular ground substance called plasma. The average blood volume is 5 or 6 liters (7% of body weight). Plasma constitutes about 55% of blood volume, cellular elements about 45%.

Plasma: Over 90% of plasma is water; the balance is made up of plasma proteins and dissolved electrolytes, hormones, antibodies, nutrients, and waste products. Plasma is isotonic (0.85% sodium chloride). Plasma plays a vital role in respiration, circulation, coagulation, temperature regulation, buffer activities and overall fluid balance.

Cardiovascular Conditions

The following cardiovascular information may be covered on your NBDE exam. Take the time to review the various conditions.

Cardiogenic Shock: heart is unable to meet the demands of the body. This can be caused by conduction system failure or heart muscle dysfunction.

Aortic insufficiency: Heart valve disease that prevents the aortic valve from closing completely. Backflow of blood into the left ventricle.

Aortic aneurysm: Expansion of the blood vessel wall often identified in the thoracic region.

Hypovolemic shock: Poor blood volume prevents the heart from pumping enough blood to the body.

Cardiogenic shock: Enough blood is available, however the heart is unable to move the blood in an effective manner.

Myocarditis: inflammation of the heart muscle.

Heart valve infection: endocarditis (inflammation), probable valvular heart disease. Can be caused by fungi or bacteria.

Pericarditis: Inflammation of the pericardium.

Arrhythmias: Irregular heart beats and rhythms disorder

Arteriosclerosis: hardening of the arteries.

Cardiomyopathy- poor hear pumping and weakness of the myocardium.

Wave Review

ST segment:	ventricles depolarized
P wave:	atrial depolarization
PR segment:	AV node conduction
QRS complex:	ventricular depolarization
U wave:	hypokalemia creates a U wave
T wave:	ventricular repolarization

Endocrine Review

Hypothyroidism: Poor production of thyroid hormone:
Primary- Thyroid cannot meet the demands of the pituitary gland.
Secondary- No stimulation of the thyroid by the pituitary gland.

Hyperthyroidism: excessive production of thyroid hormone.

Causes:
Iodine overdose
Thyroid hormone overdose
Graves' disease (key)
Tumors affecting the reproductive system

Congenital adrenal hyperplasia: Excessive production of androgen and low levels of aldosterone and cortisol. (Genetically inherited disorder). Different forms of this disorder that affect males and females differently.

Causes: Adrenal gland enzyme deficit causes cortisol and aldosterone to not be produced. Causing male sex characteristics to be expressed prematurely in boys and found in girls.

Primary/Secondary Hyperaldosteronism
Primary Hyperaldosteronism: problem within the adrenal gland causing excessive production of aldosterone.
Secondary Hyperaldosteronism: problem found elsewhere causing excessive production of aldosterone.

Cushing's syndrome: Abnormal production of ACTH which in turn causes elevated cortisol levels.

Diabetic ketoacidosis: increased levels of ketones due to a lack of glucose.

Causes: Insufficient insulin causing ketone production which end up in the urine. More common in type I vs. type 2 DM.

T3/T4 Review
Both are stimulated by TSH release from the Pituitary gland
T4 control basal metabolic rate
T4 becomes T3 within cells. (T3) Active form.
Hyperthyroidism- T3 increased, T4 normal- (in many cases)

Lymphocytic thyroiditis: Hyperthyroidism leading to hypothyroidism and then normal levels.

Graves' disease: most commonly linked to hyperthyroidism, and is an autoimmune disease. Exophthalmos may be noted (protruding eyeballs). Excessive production of thyroid hormones.

Type I diabetes (Juvenile onset diabetes)
Causes: Poor insulin production from the beta cells of the pancreas. Excessive levels of glucose in the blood stream that cannot be used due to the lack of insulin. Moreover, the patient continues to experience hunger, due to the cells not getting the fuel that they need. After 7-10 years the beta cells are completely destroyed in many cases.

Type II diabetes
The body does not respond appropriately to the insulin that is present. Insulin resistance is present in Type II diabetes. Results in hyperglycemia.

Risk factors for Type II Diabetes:
Obesity
Limited exercise individuals
Race-Minorities have a higher distribution
Elevated Cholesterol levels
Htn

Diabetes Risk Factors:

Bad diet
Htn
Weight distribution around the waist/overweight.
Certain minority groups
History of diabetes in your family
Poor exercise program
Elevated triglyceride levels

Genetics and Cell Biology

Molecular genetics. DNA: double-helix structure, its roles as template in nucleic acid synthesis.

Nucleotides: Types and three structural components of DNA and RNA; base-pairing.

Protein Synthesis. Sequence of events from transcription to translation; the roles of mRNA, tRNA, amino acid and growing peptide chain, and the ribosome. Diversity and protein functions.

Enzymes. Catalytic function and universality of. General principles of enzyme action: active site:, specificity. Regulatory enzymes and feedback inhibition. Knowledge of Michaelis-Menten kinetics (e.g., K_m) is *not* required

Metabolism. ATP as universal energy source. Glycolysis, Krebs cycle, and electron-transport chain: important steps, intracellular location, sites and amounts of ATP and CO^2 production, O^2 consumption.

Prokaryotes. Defining characteristics. Viruses: protein-DNA structure; life cycle (lytic and lysogenic); as obligate intracellular parasites; bacteriophage. Bacteria: classification by shape (e.g., cocci, bacilli, spirochetes, rickettsians). Importance of mutation, transformation, transduction.

Eucaryotes. Defining characteristics. Function and essential structure of important organelles and inclusions, such as mitochondria, ribosomes, nucleus, nuclear and cell membranes. Mitosis: stages of, principles of, associates structures. The only thing that should be known about fungi is their characteristic life cycle.

Organismal Biology

Embryology and Reproduction. Meiosis and principles of sexual reproduction. Crude understanding of male and female sexual anatomy and physiology. Fertilization of egg and subsequent developmental stages (zygote, morula, blastula, gastula, neurula). The three primary germ layers and the organs each gives rise to. Basic anatomy of the early embryo. Induction and differentiation: prototypical example – development of the vertebrate eye.

Respiration and Renal Function. Lungs as gas exchangers (of O^2, CO^2). The kidneys as excretory organs (of urea, bicarbonate, drugs, etc.) and as reabsorbing organs (e.g., of glucose, water, sodium). The glomerulus, nephron, loop of Henle.

Circulation. Basic anatomy of the heart and great vessels. Functions of arteries, arterioles, capillaries, venules, and veins. Lymphatic system: function; drainage.

Thermoregulation: counter-current heat exchange mechanism; importance of increased or decreased blood flow to the skin.

Muscle and Bone. Principles of muscle action: actinmyosin contraction, role of O^2 and lactic acid production, utilization of glucose and creatine phosphate. Characteristics of smooth, striated (voluntary), and cardiac muscle. Bone: cellular components and inorganic matrix; cartilage and organic matrix. Haversian canals. Tendons and ligaments.

Nervous System. The neuron: dendrites, cell body, axon, resting potential, impulse propagation, sodium potassium transfers. Autonomic nervous system, central vs. peripheral nervous systems, afferent vs. efferent nerves vs. interneurons. The reflex arc. Basic functions of the medulla, cerebellum, and cerebrum. The neuromuscular junction.

Endocrine System. The major glands and their hormones. The feedback loop. Special emphasis is on the sex hormones, insulin, epinephrine, antidiuretic hormone (ADH), thyroid hormone. Connection between the hypothalamus and the pituitary gland.

Digestion. Major digestive events occurring in the mouth, stomach, small intestine, and large intestine. The portal vein, liver, bile, and gall bladder. Pancreatic digestive enzymes. Villi and microvilli.

The Gene, Alleles, and Mandelian Principles. Genetic crosses, pedigree analysis. Dominance, co-dominance, sex-linkage, heterozygosity, pleitropy. Mechanism and significance of crossovers. Assumptions necessary for the Hardy-Weinberg equilibrium
(but not the Hardy-Weinberg formula)

Animal and Human behavior. Imprinting, reflex, ritual, conditioned behavior, learning, habit, insight, etc. Territoriality, competition, dominance, aggression, courtship. Predation, symbiosis, mutualism, commensalisms, parasitism, saprophytism.

Evolution. Darwinian principles (survival of the fittest); definition of fitness. Lamarckian inheritance. Evolutionary mechanisms such as speciation, radiation, extinction, convergence, divergence. Nomenclature of taxonomy (kingdom, phylum, class, order, family, genus, species) and Linnaean nomenclature. Basic comparative anatomy and general evolutionary trends in body structure. Homology and analogy (with regard to organs).

The Cell- Its Structures and Function

The cell is the basic unit of structure and function and basis of all life; all cells come from preexisting cells.

Size

Most cells are between 10 and 100μ (microns) in diameter. Measurements are made utilizing the following units:
   1 cm= 10mm
   1 mm= 1000μ
   1μ= 10,000Å (angstrom units)

Average sizes of structures may be listed as follows:
Cells about 10μ   (100,000 Å)
Mitochondria about 1μ   (10,000 Å)
Bacteria about 1μ   (10,000 Å)
Viruses about 0.1μ   (1,000 Å)
Macromolecules about 0.01μ   (100 Å)
Molecules about 0.001μ   (10 Å)
Hydrogen ion about 0.0001μ   (1 Å)

Resolution is commonly defined as the ability to discriminate two points and visualize them as two points, even though they are extremely close together. With the unaided eye these two points might appear as one point. The resolution is dependent on the wavelength of the light source and can be calculated to be about one-half the wavelength.

Examples of resolving power are:
Human eye about 0.1 mm (100μ)
Light microscope about 0.2μ (2000 Å)
Electron microscope about 2-5 Å

Composition of Protoplasm

Protoplasm is made up mainly of proteins, carbohydrates, fats, salts and water; its average elemental composition is:

Oxygen 75 + %
Carbon 10+%
Hydrogen 10+%
Nitrogen 2+%
Sulfur about 0.2%
Phosphorus about 0.3%
Potassium 0.3%
Chlorine about 0.1%
Less than 0.1% - Sodium, calcium, magnesium, iron, etc.

Properties of the Cell and Protoplasm

Irritability
1. Conductivity
2. Respiration
3. Absorption
4. Secretion
5. Excretion
6. Growth
7. Reproduction
8. Metabolism

Components of a typical Cell

Cells are commonly recognized as having two major compartments: **_Cytoplasm_** which includes all components within the cell membrane but outside of the nucleus and **_nucleoplasm_** which includes everything within the nuclear membrane.

Cell Membrane: The cell membrane, or unit membrane, usually is about 75-100 Å thick; it is a trilaminar structure. As described by Danielli and Davson (1935), two protein layers sandwich a bimolecular lipid layer.
The cell membrane:
Provides for a boundary resulting in a controlled environment.
It is a relatively watertight barrier.
Maintains a constant composition and environment resulting in homeostasis.
Is semipermiable; only certain types of molecules are allowed to pass.
Is composed mainly of proteins, lipids, and carbohydrates; the major types of lipids found in nature are fats, phospholipids, and steroids.

Structure. Electron microscopy suggests that the central region of the membrane consists of two layers of lipid molecules, mainly phospholipids and steroids. Each layer is thought to be one molecule thick. The phospholipids molecules are fairly long and have two functional poles: one exhibits lipid properties (it exhibits hydrophobic properties, repelling water); the other exhibits polar properties (it has a tendency to dissolve water, and exhibits hydrophilic properties). The hydrophobic ends of both layers of lipid molecules associate with each other since they have affinity for one another. The hydrophilic portions face toward the protein layers; parts of proteins associate readily with water.
Electron microscopy substantiates that there is a light central layer surrounded by two denser layers. The two denser layers are thought to represent the proteins and hydrophilic portions of the lipid molecules.

Activities. The plasma membrane is semi-permeable. It controls the passage of materials into and out of the cell. The movement of materials into and out of the cell is called *transport.*

There are two types of transport—passive, or transport that does not require the cells energy, and active, which does require the energy expenditure.
There are two types of passive transport—diffusion and osmosis.
In *diffusion* molecules pass from an area of higher concentration to that of lower concentration until the concentrations are equal on both sides of the membrane. Diffusion, in other words, follows the concentration gradient.

Osmosis is the movement of water across the semi-permeable membrane. Water will pass into a more concentrated solution and this passage of water will equalize the concentration of dissolved substances on each side of the membrane so that equilibrium is theoretically achieved.

Equilibrium implies an equal number of molecules of all dissolved material per unit volume on each side of the membrane compartment; the same applies to the concentration of each individual diffusible component.

Gases pass through the cell membrane with ease. Water and small molecules pass more readily than large molecules and lipid soluble materials enter the cell easier than non lipid soluble substances.

Active transport requires the cell to expand energy to allow materials to pass through the membrane. (Also called uphill transport, energy dependent transport can operate against concentration gradients.) Electrical charge has also to be considered. The inside of the cell is usually electrically negative in comparison to the outside environment.

In active transport, materials enter the cell in membrane-bound vesicles, formed by the membrane. This process is known collectively as *endocytosis.* When it involves solid material we speak of *phagocytosis;* liquid materials enters via *pinocytosis.* The process of expulsion of material is known as *exocytosis.*

Special Sites. To amplify the complexities of the cell membrane some general statements are in order at this point.

Cells must be held together and specialized structures are required. Adjacent cell membranes interdigitate and intercellular cement is utilized.

A *desmosome* is a specialized area of connection between adjacent cellular membranes (macula adherens).

A terminal bar is a dense area surrounding the apical cellular surface. It includes the tight junction (zona occludens) and the loose junction (zona adherens).

Layers of material (probably mucopolysaccharide) secreted by the cell are found on the surface of the cell. The most prominent layer is the *basement membrane,* or *basal lamina.*

The thick cellulose cell wall of plants falls within the above category. These structures are boundaries and must be traversed by material entering and leaving the cell.

Intercellular Space

Cells are usually separated by a space of about 100-200 Å. Only at specialized contact points do cells appose each other. The space is filled mainly by a matrix of proteins and polysaccharides which function in cementing cells to one another.

Some cells possess special extracellular polysaccharide substances: cartilage is rich in chrondroitin sulfate; joints have large amounts of hyaluronic acid; and cell walls of plants are composed largely of cellulose.

Cytoplasmic matrix

The cytoplasm of a cell appears homogeneous, translucent, and structureless; the homogeneous mass, which is also called cell-sap or hyaloplasm, contains inorganic substances and organic compounds of varying molecular sizes. The more peripheral layer of this matrix is also known as ectoplasm (plasmagel). It appears more rigid and seems to lack granules completely.

Cellular Inclusions

These may be composed of proteins, fats, carbohydrates, granules, pigments, and crystals.
   a) *Secretion granules (products of cell activity)*. These are usually membrane-bound products that await extrusion by the cell (exocrine secretion into ducts or endocrine secretion into the extracellular space and capillaries).Release of secretory product from the cells is via exocytosis. Under the general term endocytosis (taking into the cell), are the more specific terms, pinocytosis (taking in of fluid) and phagocytosis (taking in of solids).
   b) *Lipid droplets*. These are globular accumulations synthesized by the cell. During periods of need they may serve as a source of energy.
   c) *Glycogen granules*. These are small spherical units synthesized by the cell. They serve as storage reservoirs of carbohydrates.
   d) *Pigment granules*. These may be of two types: endogenous pigments derived from cell metabolismor exogenous pigments taken in by the cell. Hemosiderin, is an example of an exogenous pigment, while the lipochromes and the melanins are endogenous in nature.
   e) *Vacuoles*. Under this general term may be classified any membrane-bound globular structure.
   f) *Plastids*. The plastids are composed of leucoplasts, chromoplasts and chloroplasts. Leucoplasts resemble chloroplasts but have no chlorophyll; they manufacture starch, oil and protein. Chromoplasts possess pigments and are responsible for the color of flower petals. Chloroplastspossess chlorophyll, which is capable of capturing light energy to produce Glucose from CO^2 and H^2O.

Mitochondria

Mitochondria are the best known of the cellular organelles. They had been described during the 19th century, notably by Kollicker and Fleming. Altman, using Janus green, was able to stain them in 1890. Structually, the mitochondrion is composed of an outer trilaminar membrane and an inner trilaminar membrane; the inner one forms folds which are known as *cristae*. The space between the two membranes is about 6-10 nm wide.

Mitochondria as a whole and specifically the cristae vary in size, shape and number not only in different cells but also in the same cell depending on its functional state. Mitochondria are present in greater numbers in cells exhibiting high levels of activity and having more energy requirements. Muscle and grandular tissues fall in the above category.
DNA has been found in the mitochondria of animals and the chloroplasts of plants. Mitochondria are capable of division and are not generated *de novo.*
Granules have been observed in the mitochondria Matrix. Their identity is in question, however; some believe they might be reservoirs of calcium and other divalent ions. Phosphate is taken up with Ca^{2+} and calcium phosphate deposit may be the end result.

Mitochondria are the biochemical power plants of the cell. They recover energy from food stuffs (via krebs cycle, or citric acid cycle; tricarboxylic acid cycle and the respiratory chain) and convert it via phosphorylation into adenosine triphosphate (ATP). In this manner they produce the energy necessary for the metabolic processes.

Enzymes. The organization of enzymes and coenzymes(especially enzymes involved in odidative phosphorylation) in the cristae appears to be highly specific facilitating an orderly and proper sequence of reactions.
Enzymes concerned with the Krebs cycle are presumed to be either free in the mitochondrial matrix (internal medium) or loosely bound to the membranes since they are readily recovered when mitochondria are disrupted. The electron transport and oxidative phosphorylation seem to be coupled.
Enzymes then are associated with the outer membrane, the inner membrane, the space between the outer and inner membranes, and the matrix.

DNA and protein Synthesis. Most extranuclear DNA, if not all, can be found in mitochondria (and in plants in the chloroplast). Thereis evidence that proteins are synthesized in mitochondria under direction of mitochondrial DNA. In biochemical preparations of mitochondria the synthesizing enzymes necessary for RNA and proteins
Have been isolated.However, there is also considerable documentation that the code for the enzymes involved in oxidative phosphorylation originates in nuclear DNA. Therefore, it must be assumed that mitochondrial DNA is involved only in the partial coding of the proteins manufactured in the organelle.

Krebs Cycle. Mitochondria are involved in the Krebs citric acid cycle in which organic acids are oxidized to CO^2. In each successive step oxidation of a single carbon of the chain takes place and each reaction requires a different enzyme. The ATP produced is a small molecule and can diffuse out of the mitochondrion into the cytoplasm and participate in the endothermic reactions of the cell.

Endoplasmic Reticulum (ER)

This cellular organelle was first described using phase microscopy by Porter, Claude and Fallam in 1945. It is an extensive network of interconnecting channels. The endoplasmic reticular membranes are unit membranes (triminar). When ribosomes line the outer surface it is designated as *rough endoplasmic reticulum* (RER). The primary form of this organelle is the rough variety. The smooth is derived from the rough due to loss of ribosomes. The amount of each depends on the cell type and the cellular activity.

The RER is the synthetic machinery of the cell. It is mainly concerned with protein synthesis.

The Golgi Complex

This structure was discovered by Camillo Golgi in 1898. All eukaryotic cells, except for the red blood cell, possess a Golgi apparatus. Generally speaking the Golgi complex is prominent in glandular cells and is thought to function in the production, concentration packaging, and transportation of secretory material. IN summary one can link the Golgi complex to: secretion, membrane biogenesis, lysosome formation, membrane recycling, hormone modulation.

Lysosome

Lysosomes are described as containing proteolytic enzymes (hydrolases).Lysosomes contain acid phosphatase and other hydrolytic enzymes.. These enzymes are enclosed by a membrane and are released when needed into the cell or into phagocytic vesicles.

Lysosomal enzymes have the capacity to hydrolyze all classes of macromolecules.

A generalized list of substrates acted upon by respective enzymes is given bellow:

Lipids by lipases and phospholipases;
Proteins by proteases or peptidases;
Polysaccharides by glycosidases;
Nucleic acids by nucleases;

Phosphates (organic-linked) by phosphatases;
Sulphates (organic-linked) by sulfatases.

Peroxisomes

Peroxisomes are found in virtually all mammalian cell types and probably arise from swellings of the endoplasmic Reticulum. These structures are often smaller than lysosomes. These enzymes they possess are active in the production of hydrogen peroxide (urate oxidase, D-amino acid oxidase, α-hydroxyacid oxidase), and one functions in destroying hydrogen peroxide (catalase). The peroxisomes function in purine catabolism and in the degradation of nucleic acids.

Nucleus

The nucleus was first described by Robert Brown in 1831. The nucleus is surrounded by a double layer of the typical trilaminar membrane which is pierced by small pores. The pores measure about 50-80 nm in diameter.The pores allow and serve in the interchange of nuclear and cytoplasmic material.

Aproximate composition of the nucleus:
80% protein, 15% DNA, 5% RNA, 3% lipid.

Functions: Simply speaking, the nucleus controls the metabolic aspects of the cell and is responsible for its structural integrity, function, survival and passage of the hereditary material to the next generation.

DNA Structure, *DNA*-deoxyribonucleic acid – is a nucleic acid. A nucleic acid is a polymer of nucleotides. The combination of *purine* or *pyrimidine* base, a sugar, and phosphoric acid is called a *nucleotide*. *Deoxyrobose* is the sugar in DNA; ribose is the other nucleic acid, ribonucleic acid, or RNA.

DNA molecules are composed of two nucleotide strands coiled together in a double helix. Watson and Crick (1953) proposed a double helix model of DNA. The two strands consist of sugar-phosphate backbones which are connected by pairs of bases.All DNA nucleotides consist of a 5-carbon sugar (deoxyribose) with a phosphate group attached at one end and a nitrogen-containing ring compound (the base) at the other. The nitrogenous bases are: adenine and guanine (*purines*) and thymine, cytosine, and uracil (*pyrimidines*). In DNA they pair specifically in the following manner:

Adenine and Thymine ....Guanine and Cytosine.

RNA pair as follows:
Adenine and Uracil ....Guanine and Cyrosine.

The paired bases are held together by hydrogen bonds.

Characteristics of DNA and RNA

DNA
Double stranded
Sugar-deoxyribose
Base- thymine

RNA
Single stranded (mainly)
Sugar- ribose
Base- uracil

DNA determines and acts as a template for RNA synthesis. With the help of a transcription enzyme (RNA polymerase) a complementary RNA strand is produced. The base pairings are as follows:
DNA   T-thymine, C-cytosine
RNA   A-adenine, G-guanine.

Once RNA has been manufactured in the nucleus it moves fairly quickly into the cytoplasm.

Messenger RNA (mRNA) from the nucleus brings the coded message for protein synthesis to ribosomal RNA (rRNA). Ribosomal RNA imparts the message to *transfer RNA* (Trna), which carries the specific amino acids coded for to the ribosomes, where protein synthesis is carried out.

Chromatin. The survivor of the cell, organism, and species depends upon the chromatin material in the nucleus. Chromatin is DNA combined with protein, and stains with basic dyes. During the interphase of the cell cycle some chromosomes are visualized as tight coils and are referred to as *heterochromatin*.

Ribosomes and Polysomes: Ribosomes may be free or attached to the membranes of the endoplasmic Reticulum, which is then designated as rough ER. Ribosomes are the sites of protein synthesis in the cell. If ribosomes appear in clusters (rosettes) in the cytoplasm, they are commonly termed *polyribosomes* or *polysomes*.

Ribosomes possess RNA known as ribosomal RNA (rRNA) and both rRNA and messenger RNA (mRNA) are produced on DNA templates in the nucleus.

Microtubules: These structures are usually associated with centrioles and basal bodies. They are also present in the cytoplasm of various cells, in particular the axons of neurons. Microtubules apparently function in the maintenance of the structural integrity (shape and rigidity) of the cell. Transport of material and movement of cilia and flagella are also ascribed to these organelles.

Microfilaments: These structures are prominent in the microvilli of the absorptive cells of the intestines. They have been shown to be associated with the regions of the terminal web and the desmosome.

Centrioles, Cilia and Flagella: The centrioles are self-reproducing organelles that play an important role in the separation of the chromosomes during mitosis. Before division of the cell the centriole splits into two and the daughter centrioles migrate to opposite sides of the nucleus. The form the center of the *spindle* and *aster* configuration during cell division.

Organelles almost identical in structure to the centriole are the basal bodies of cilia and flagella. The structure and function of cilia and flagella are similar. They, like the centriole, have nine (9) sets of tubules arranged in a peripheral cylinder; the sets, however, are doublets, not triplets. And unlike centrioles, cilia and flagella have an additional pair of central tubules. Therefore, we can summarize the arrangement in centrioles as 9 + 0-, and in cilia and flagella as 9 + 2.

Cell Division – Mitosis

For purposes of convenience, mitosis is divided into prophase, metaphase, anaphase, and telophase; the process, however, is a continuous one. The major events during the phases are:

1. *Prophase:* Chromosomes become distinct and nucleolus (nucleoli) disappear(s); centriole(s) and asters and spindle appear; nuclear membrane disappears.

2. *Metaphase*: Chromosomes move to the equator of the cell and duplicate.

3. Anaphase: The two chromatids split apart and start migration toward the poles of the spindle; the spindle loses its definition.

4. *Telophase:* Chromosomes lengthen and become less distinct; nucleoli reappear. The next period of growth and rest is known as *interphase*.

5. *Interphase:* Cell growth; protein synthesis; DNA synthesis; chromosome duplication.

Methods of Examining the Cell

1. Histological Methods:

    a. *Microscopy*
    b. *Stains*

2. Histochemical Methods: Tissues are composed of various chemicals such as proteins, carbohydrates, lipids, inorganic salts and miscellaneous substances, and various tests are used to detect these chemicals.

Examples:

Proteins (with tyrosine) – yellow color;
1) Enzymes – various tests for phosphatases, lipases, oxidases, exterases, and dehydrogenases;
2) Carbohydrates – glycogen by periodic acid Schiff (PAS) test results in a magenta or purple color; glycolproteins give a positive PAS magenta color. Basal laminae and reticular fibers are strongly PAS positive;
3) Lipids – Sudan dyes or osmic acid;
4) Nucleic acids – Feulgen reaction is specific for DNA, but not for RNA, which can be detected by ribonuclease. Both DNA and RNA are basophilic (because they are both acids).

3. Fixation: The fixative must modify the cell to resist further treatments and also to make further treatments possible. Fixatives may be classified as either coagulant or non-coagulant. Examples of each are:

1) *coagulant:* methanol, ethanol, acetone, nitric acid, hydrochloric acid, picric acid, trichloroacetic acid and mercuric chloride.
2) *non*-coagulant: formaldehyde, glutaraldehyde, osmium tetroxide, potassium dichromate, acetic acid, and potassium permanganate.

Fixatives can also be sub classified into two categories. The following are examples:

1) *additive:* osmium tetroxide, formaldehyde, and glutaraldehyde.
2) *Non-additive:* methanol, ethanol, and acetone.

1. **Method of Preparation**

   1) *Fixation*
   2) *Dehydration*
   3) *Embedding*
   4) *Sectioning*
   5) *Staining*

Polygenic Traits

The distribution of individuals with different trait values for polygenic (quantitative) traits in a population is typically a bell-shaped curve, as shown here:

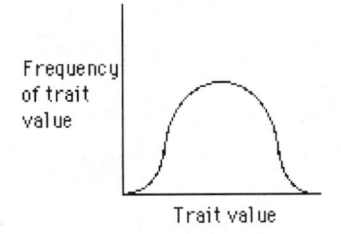

There are three main ways selection could act on a population, given a distribution of traits such as this. These are:

1. **Directional selection:** the situation in which one extreme form of the trait has highest fitness.

2. **Stabilizing selection:** the situation in which the average form of the trait has higher fitness than does either extreme.

3. **Disruptive selection:** the situation in which both extreme forms of the trait have higher fitness than does the average.

The results of selection on quantitative traits generally makes sense -- the forms that have highest fitness become most common. As shown, **directional selection** results in a change in the mean value of the trait toward the form that has highest fitness. **Stabilizing selection** results in the loss of the extreme forms of the trait; this means there is a decrease in genetic variation -- eventually, genetic variation may be lost, as all individuals will have the alleles for the highest fitness, average, trait value. At this point, any phenotypic variation would depend on direct environmental effects rather than on genetic differences among individuals, and the heritability of the trait would be zero, or at least very low. **Disruptive selection** results in an increase in both extremes and a loss of intermediate forms.

Over a long period of time **directional selection** will result in a shift in the frequency of individuals with different traits until the average form has highest fitness. At this point, the situation becomes one of stabilizing selection, and the extreme forms of the trait will be lost. So directional selection eventually will lead to a situation where genetic variation will be lost (heritability will become zero) and all individuals will have the alleles for the highest fitness form of the trait.

Major Hormones

Growth hormone- major stimulus of postnatal growth: Induces precursor cells to differentiate and secrete insulin-like growth factor I which stimulates cell division, stimulates protein synthesis

Insulin-stimulates fetal growth, stimulates postnatal growth by stimulating secretion of IGF-1, stimulates protein synthesis

Thyroid hormones-permissive for growth hormone's secretion and actions, permissive for development of the central nervous system

Testosterone-stimulates growth at puberty, in large part by stimulating the secretion of growth hormone, causes eventual epiphyseal closure, stimulates protein synthesis
Estrogen-stimulates the secretion of growth hormone at puberty, causes eventual epiphyseal closure
Cortisol-inhibits growth, stimulates protein catabolism

Gland Review

Sublingual- On each side underneath the tongue in the floor of the mouth, Multiple separate ducts, Smallest of the salivary glands

Submandibular- Posterior portion of the mandible, lingual to the mandibular incisors, Opens under the tongue close to the frenum, Secretes watery fluid with some mucus. More viscous (thick) than parotid secretion

Parotid- Inside cheek opposit maxillary second molars, Parotid ducts go through the buccinator muscles and enter the mouth opposite maxillary second molars, Largest of the salivary glands. Secretes clear watery fluid

Dental Anatomy

Key Terms

Enamel
The hardest calcified tissue in the body, it consists of enamel rods that are brittle and subject to disintegration and breakage by acid produced on the tooth surface by bacteria.

Dentin
Pain stimuli are transmitted through microscopic tubules found in dentin. Each tubule contains a nerve fiber that penetrates the porous dentin.

Pulp Chamber
This is the terminating point of blood vessels and nerves. Stimuli are transmitted and received by the pulp.

Root
The root is the portion of the tooth in the alveolar bone. It is covered by a coat of material similar to bone called cementum.

Root Apex
The entrance point of the nerve, blood vessels and connective tissue that constitutes the pulp.

The Basics

Teeth are numbered in the following manner. As you can see, the mouth is divided into 4 quadrants, with 8 teeth per quadrant.

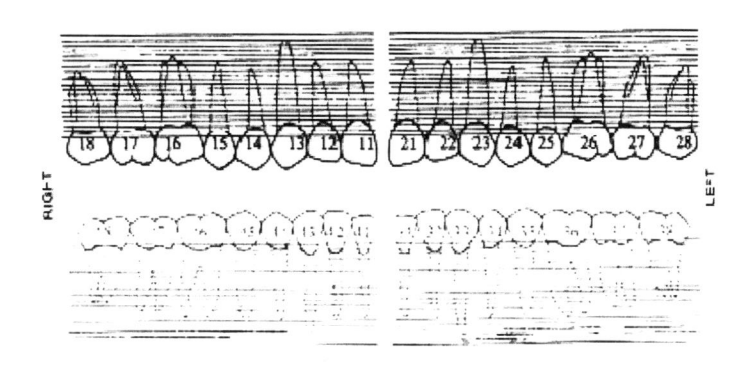

Teeth are named in the following manner:

Incisors - The four front teeth, known as the biting edge of the anterior teeth
Cuspids - Teeth next to the incisors. One tooth per quadrant, primarily used in tearing/ripping food
Premolars - Two teeth per quadrant. In between the molars and the cuspids
Molars - The back twelve teeth, used to chew. Three teeth per quadrant
Buccal - Surface of tooth adjacent to the cheek. Describes the facial surface for premolars and molars
Labial - Lip/front part of the facial surface for incisors and canines
Facial - Outer surface of teeth (labial + buccal)
Lingual - Surface of tooth adjacent to the tongue
Distal - Surface of the tooth away from the midline
Mesial - Surface of the tooth towards the midline
Occlusal - The biting surface of posterior teeth
Therefore, individual cusps are named in the following manner:
Mesiobuccal, Mesiolingual, Distobuccal and Distolingual

Secondary teeth - There are a total of 32 secondary teeth. (8 incisors, 4 cuspids, 8 premolars and 12 molars). Secondary molars erupt behind primary molars. The first secondary tooth to erupt is the first molar, and it usually does so around 6 years of age. The 3rd molar is the last to erupt and comes in around the age of 21 years All other teeth are usually present by the age of 14 years.

Primary teeth differ from secondary teeth in many ways. Specifically, there are a total of 20 primary teeth (8 incisors, 4 cuspids and 8 molars). No premolars are developed at this time. Incisors are the first primary teeth to erupt and usually do so between 6-9 months The last teeth usually grow in by 24 months

Jaws and Dental Arches

The teeth are arranged in upper and lower arches. Those of the upper are called maxillary; those of the lower are mandibular.

A. The maxilla is actually two bones forming the upper jaw; they are rigidly attached to the skull.

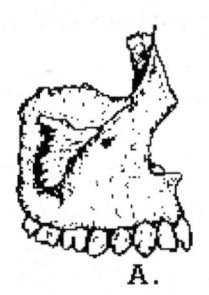

B. The mandible is a horseshoe shaped bone which articulates with the skull by way of the temporomandibular joint the TMJ.

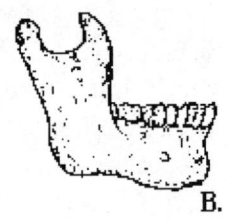

C. The dental arches, the individual row of teeth forming a tooth row attached to their respective jaw bones have a distinctive shape known as a catenary arch.

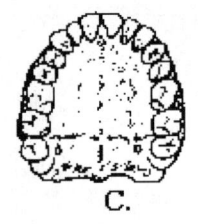

Dentition is a term that describes all of the upper and lower teeth collectively. Clinically, there are three dentitions.

A. The primary dentition consists of 20 teeth in all: ten upper and ten lower teeth. Primary teeth may also be called 'baby' teeth, deciduous, 'milk', or lacteal teeth. Primary teeth begin to appear at about age six months and are entirely replaced by about ages 12 - 13.

B. The mixed dentition is composed of both primary and permanent teeth. It commences with the eruption of the first of the permanent teeth at about age six, and ends with the loss of the last of the deciduous teeth at about the age of 12-13 years

C. The permanent dentition is composed of 32 teeth in all, 16 upper and 16 lower. Half of a dental arch (primary or permanent) is called a quadrant. The permanent teeth that replace deciduous teeth are call succedaneous teeth. (Succedaneous means literally, to replace. In dental science, permanent teeth that replace deciduous teeth are called successional teeth. Permanent molars, which replace nothing are called accessional teeth.)

D. Types of dentitions:
1. Diphyodont. Most mammals--humans included--typically develope and erupt into their jaws two generations of teeth. The term literally means "two generations of teeth."
2. Monophyodont. Some mammals--such as the manatee, seals, and walruses have only a single generation of teeth.
3. Polyphyodont. Most reptiles and fishes develop a lifetime of generations of successional teeth--as if on a conveyer belt. Such teeth have a brief functional life and are anatomically simple in design.
4. Homodont. In many vertebrates, all of the teeth in the jaw are alike. They differ from each other only in size. The alligator is an example of homodontism.
5. Heterodont. Most mammals, humans included, develop distinctive classes of teeth that are regionally specialized. We will discuss classes of teeth in the next unit.
6. Anodontia is the developmental absence of teeth. Among mammals, the whalebone whale and the anteater are toothless; their ancestors had teeth. In humans, anodontia is a pathological condition. Partial anodontia is one or a few teeth missing.

Classes of Teeth

A. Anterior teeth
1. Incisors: Four uppers and four lowers. There are central incisors and lateral incisors. These function in cutting food, articulating speech, appearance, and for support of the lips.
2. Canines: Two upper and two lower. In dogs and cats, the long canine teeth are used for catching food, tearing the food, and for defense. In some primates, I large canines are used in threatening gestures. In humans, they function along with the incisors for support of the lips, cutting or shearing of food, and as guideposts in occlusion. In traditional re storative dentistry, they are the cornerstones of the dental arch.

B. Posterior teeth (Cheek Teeth)
1. Premolars: Also known as bicuspids. They are four number in the upper arch and four in number thelo arch. They are designated as first or second bicuspi their order in the dental arch. They function wi molars in the mastication of food and in maintaini vertical dimension of the face.
2. Molars: There are six upper and six lower, designated as first, second, or third. Permanent molars are important in the chewing and grinding of food, and in maintaining the vertical dimension. Important: Upper molars have three roots and low molars have two roots.

Dental Formula, Dental Notation, Universal Numbering System

A. Dental Formula. The dental formula expresses the type and number of teeth per side. It is used by comparative anatomists and zoologists. It appears on National Boards, our exams, and scholarly articles.

1. Primary teeth.

It is said as: incisors, two upper and two lower; canines, one upper and one lower; molars two upper and two lower equals ten per side.

$$I\frac{2}{2} - C\frac{1}{1} - M\frac{2}{2} = 10$$

2. Permanent teeth.

It is said as: incisors, two upper and two lower; canines, one upper and one lower; premolars, two upper and two lower; and molars, three upper and three lower. Comment: You won't use it clinically, but you should be aware of it.

$$I\frac{2}{2} - C\frac{1}{1} - Pm\frac{2}{2} - M\frac{3}{3} = 16$$

B. Dental Notation: Several systems of dental notation have been used over the years. Many orthodontists, for example, retain an older system that uses just numbers or letters for the teeth with lines or brackets to designate upper or lower.

C. The Universal Numbering System. The rules are as follows:

1. Permanent teeth are designated by number, beginning with the last tooth on the upper right side, going on to the last tooth on the left side, then lower left to lower right. There are thirty-two pemanent teeth, correct?

$$R \frac{1 \quad\quad 8\ 9 \quad\quad 16}{32 \quad\quad 25\ 24 \quad\quad 17} L$$

2. Deciduous teeth are designated by letter, beginning with the last tooth on the upper right side and proceeding in clockwise fashion as described above We will cover this again in our unit on deciduous teeth.

$$R \frac{ABCDE \quad\quad FGHIJ}{TSRQP \quad\quad ONMLK} L$$

Parts of the Tooth

A. Crown. The term can be defined in two ways.
1. The anatomical crown is covered with enamel.
2. The clinical crown is the portion of the anatomical crown that is visible clinically. It is what you see when you look in the mouth.

B. Root. The term can be defined in two ways.
1. The anatomical root is the portion of the tooth that is covered with cementum, a bone-like substance that facilitates anchorage of the tooth in its bony socket (the alveolus).
2. The clinical root is that part of the anatomical root that is actually embedded in the jaw. In a patient with advanced bone loss, the clinical root may be reduced in size.

C. Cervical line. This is the line that separates the anatomic crown from the anatomic root. It is the junction between two tissues--the enamel and the cementum. It is also called the cemento-enamel junction or simply the CEJ. This region of the tooth is also called the cervix of the tooth. The cervical line is important in your laboratory drawings.

D. Pulp cavity. This is the space in the tooth that in life contains the pulp or 'nerve' of the tooth. In your specimens, the pulp will be withered or absent. It has a coronal (crown) portion and a radicular (root) portion, usually called the rooth canal.

Dental Tissues

A. Enamel. The protective outer surface of the anatomic crown. It is 96% mineral and is the hardest tissue in the body.
B. Dentin. Located in both the crown and root, it makes up the bulk of the tooth beneath the enamel and cementum. It lines the pulp cavity.
C. Cementum. This substance covers the surface of the anatomic root.
D. Pulp. The central, innermost portion of the tooth. It has formative, sensory, nutritive, and functions during the life of the tooth.

Points of Reference

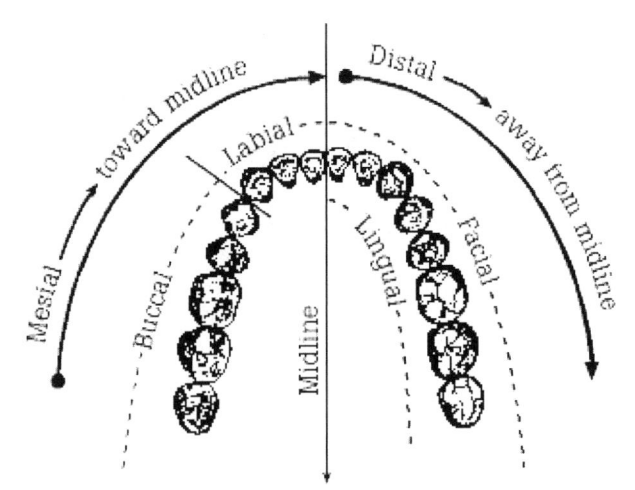

Median sagittal plane: the imaginary plane in the center that divides right from left.
Median line: an imaginary line on that plane that bisects the dental arch at the center.
Mesial: toward the center (median) line of the dental arch.
Distal: away from the center (median) line of the dental arch.
Occlusal plane: A plane formed by the cusps of the teeth. It is often curved, as in a cylinder. We will speak often of the occlusal surface of a tooth.
Proximal: the surface of a tooth that is toward another tooth in the arch.
Mesial surface: toward the midline.
Distal surface: away from the midline.
Facial: toward the cheeks or lips.
Labial: facial surface of anterior teeth (toward the lips).
Buccal: facial surfaceof anterior teeth (toward the cheeks).
Occlusal: the biting surface; that surface that articulates with an antagonist tooth in an opposing arch.
Incisal: cutting edge of anterior teeth.
Apical: toward the apex, the tip of the root.

Dental Terminology

Cusp: a point or peak on the occlusal surface of molar and premolar teeth and on the incisal edges of canines. Wheeler's text also defines it as an elevation on the crown of a tooth making up a divisional part of the occlusal surface.
Contact: a point or area where one tooth is in contact (touching) its neighbor.
Cingulum: a bulge or elevation on the lingual surface of incisors or canines. It makes up the bulk of the cervical third of the lingual surface. Its convexity mesiodistally resembles a girdle (L. cingulum = girdle) encircling the lingual surface at the cervical.

Lobe: one of the primary centers of formation in the development of the crown of the tooth.
Mamelon: A lobe seen on anterior teeth; any one of three rounded protuberances *seen on the unworn surfaces of freshly erupted anterior teeth.*
Ridge: Any linear elevation on the surface of a tooth. It is named according to its location or form. Examples are buccal ridges, incisal ridges, marginal ridges, and so on.
Marginal ridges are those rounded borders of enamel which form the margins of the surfaces of premolars and molars, mesially and distally, and the mesial and distal margins of the incisors and canines lingually.
Triangular ridges are those ridges which descend from the tips of the cusps of molars and premolars toward the central part of the occlusal surface.
Transverse ridges are created when a buccal and lingual triangular ridge join.
Oblique ridges are seen on maxillary molars and are a companion to the distal oblique groove.
Cervical ridges are the height of contour at the gingival, on certain deciduous and permanent teeth.
Fossa: An irregular, rounded depression or concavity found on the surface of a tooth. A lingual fossa is found on the lingual surface of incisors. A central fossa is found on the occlusal surface of a molar. They are formedby the converging of ridges terminating at a central point in the bottom of a depression where there is a junction of grooves.
Pit: A small pinpoint depression located at the junction of developmental grooves or at the terminals of these groops. A central pit is found in the central fossa on the occlusal surfaces of molars where developmental grooves join. A pit is often the site of the onset ofdental caries.
Developmental groove: A sharply defined, narrow and linear depression formed during tooth development and usually separating lobes or major portions of a tooth. Major grooves are named according to their location.
A supplemental groove is also a shallow linear depression but it is usually less distinct and is more variable than a developmental groove and does not mark the junction of primary parts of a tooth.
Buccal and lingual grooves are developmental grooves found on the buccal and lingual surfaces of posterior teeth.
Tubercle: A small elevation produced by an extra formation of enamel. These occur on the marginal ridges of posterior teeth or on the cingulum of anterior teeth. These are deviations from the typical form.
Interproximal space: The triangular space between the adjacent teeth cervical to the contact point. The base of the triangle is the alveolar bone; the sides are the proximal surfaces of the adjacent teeth. Note well: the interproximal space is normally

Embrasures: When two teeth in the same arch are in contact, their curvatures adjacent to the contact areas form spillway spaces called embrasures. There are three embrasures:

(1) Facial (buccal or labial)
(2) Occlusal or incisal
(3) Lingual (Special note: there are three embrasures; the fourth potential space is the interproximal space defined above.)

(3) Lingual (Special note: there are three embrasures; the fourth potential space is the interproximal space defined above.)

Location and position

A. For purposes of description, the crowns and roots are arbitrarily divided into thirds. This is helpful in describing features such as height of contour or any other anatomic feature. A glance at the diagram to the right will clarify this for you.

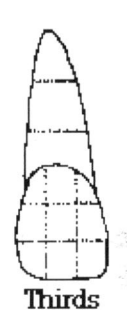

Thirds

B. The teeth present us with rounded surfaces, yet the intersection of these surfaces can clearly be described as line angles. Line angles are used as descriptive terms to indicate a position.
A line angle is the intersection of two planes. Carefully examine the diagrams at the right to clarify this concept in your mind. Line angles derive their names from the combination of the two surfaces that interesect (along a line).

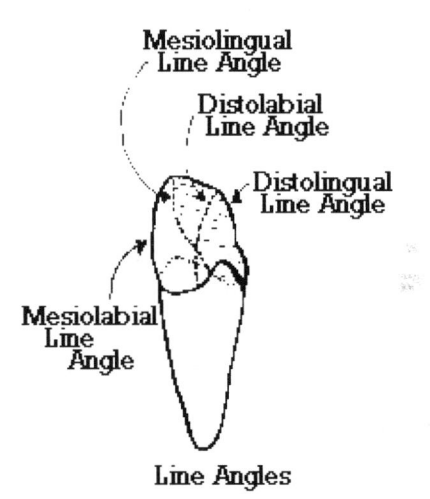

Mesiolingual Line Angle
Distolabial Line Angle
Distolingual Line Angle
Mesiolabial Line Angle

Line Angles

C. A point angle is formed by the junction of three surfaces. The point angle also derives its name from the combination of the names of the surfaces forming it. Take a look at the diagram to the right to clarify this concept in your mind.

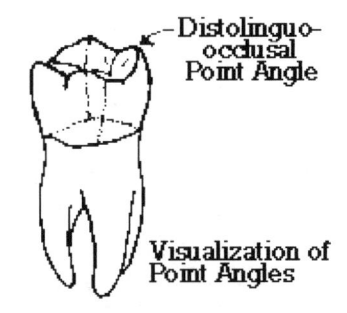

Distolinguo-occlusal Point Angle

Visualization of Point Angles

Teeth

A. Enamel

The enamel is the hard substance that covers the crown of the tooth. It is highly mineralized and is totally acellular. Enamel is the hardest substance in the body. The primary mineral component is hydroxy apatite. The susceptibility of mineral component to dissolution in an acid environment is the basis for dental decay (caries). In its mature state, it is 96% mineral.

Formation of enamel is completed before eruption of the tooth into the oral cavity. It is thickest at the cusp tips (2.0-2.6 mm) and tapers off to a knife edge at the cementoenamel junction. (CEJ).

Enamel is extremely brittle and is dependent on the underlying dentin for support. It is semitranslucent and is yellow to grayish white in appearance. Enamel is a selectively permeable membrane, allowing water and certain ions to pass via osmosis.

The fundamental morphologic unit of enamel is the enamel rod. Each is formed in increments by a single enamel forming cell, the ameoloblast. Each rod traverses uninterupted through the thickness of enamel. They number 5 to 12 million rods per crown. The rods increase in diameter (4 up to 8 microns) as they flare outward from the dentinoenamel junction.

The dentinoenamel junction is the interface between the dentin and enamel. It is the remnant of the onset of enamel formation. You will see it when you do sections of teeth in the laboratory.

Enamel formation begins at the future cusp and spreads down the cusp slope. As the ameoloblasts retreat in incremental steps, they create an artifact in the enamel called the lines of Retzius. Where these lines terminate at the tooth surface they create tiny valleys on the tooth surface that travel circumferentially around the crown known as perikymata.
(Enamel is produced in a rhythmical fashion.)

B. Dentin

This is the specialized connective tissue that makes up the bulk of the tooth, extending for almost its entire length. Dentin is hard, elastic, and is 70% mineral. Unlike enamel which is acellular, dentin has a cellular component which is retained after its formation by cells called odontoblasts. A characteristic of dentin is that it is permeated by closely packed tubules traversing its thickness and which contain cytoplasmic extensions that form dentin and maintain the dentin. When pulp of the tooth dies or is removed by the dentist, the dentin becomes brittle and is liable to fracture.

The color of dentin is yellowish white. The hardness of dentin is less than enamel but is greater than that of bone or cementum. Like enamel, it is is semipermeable to certain ions.

Each odontoblast gives rise to a cytoplasmic extension traversing the thickness of the dentin. The odontoblastic processes occupy the dentinal tubules. These processes were formerly called Tomes' fibres. There is one per odontoblast. In older persons, the dentinal tubules 'silt up' with mineralized substance. In a section, the dentin appears transparent and is called sclerotic dentin.

Dentin sensitivity in the live tooth is mediated by Tomes' fibres. One square millimeter of exposed dentin involves 30,000 odontoblasts and their corresponding Tomes' fibres. The prudent clinician, therefore, will take care not to overheat or dessicate the dentin during restorative procedures.

During dentinogenesis, odontoblasts secrete matrix in discrete increments as the odontoblasts retreat. This matrix, called predentin subsequently calcifies. Phases of mineralization remain visible in the dentin as the contour lines of Owen. These are analogous to the lines of Retzius in enamel. At birth, a neonatal line appears in the dentin of primary teeth and first permanent molars.

Dentin formation is a continuous process throughout the life of the tooth. Dentin has a reparative capability since the odontoblasts remain viable after eruption of the tooth. In response to excessive wear, caries, or irritants, dentin is laid down at an accelerated rate. This is reparative secondary dentin. Contrast this with enamel, which has no reparative capacity.

C. Dental Pulp
The dental pulp occupies the central portion of the tooth--the pulp cavity. It is a remnant of the embryologic organ for tooth development. We have already discussed one of its components--the odontoblast, a word that literally means 'tooth former.' In the adult dentition, the activity of the odontoblasts continues, producing what is called physiologic secondary dentin. Contrast this with the intermittant process of reparative secondary dentin. In time, the pulp chamber can be virtually obliterated.

The primary function of the pulp is to form dentin. The second function is nutritive: the pulp keeps the organic components of the surrounding mineralized tissue supplied with moisture and nutrients. The third function is sensory: extremes in temperature, pressure, or insult to the dentin or pulp is perceived as pain. A fourth function is protective--the formation of reparative secondary dentin.

Nerves and blood vessels access the pulp chamber via the apical foramen. Occasionally, there are accessory foramina.

D. Cementum

This is the calcified connective tissue that covers the anatomic root of the tooth. It is the least visible of the tissues to the practicing dentist, yet it serves a vital function in the support of the tooth. Cementum anchors the periodontal ligament to the root of the tooth. It is bone-like and light yellow.

Cementum is the thinnest at the cementoenamel junction and is thickest at the apex. It is laid down throughout life and resting lines can be seen in histological sections. Continous cementum deposition maintains the length of the tooth as a physiologic compensation for occlusal wear. You will occasionally see heavy accretions of cementum on the roots of teeth extracted from older patients.

This tissue is important in orthodontics: it is more resistant to resorption than alveolar bone, permitting orthodontic movement of teeth without root resorption. Histologically, there are two types of cementum: acellular which does not contain cells, and cellular which contains entrapped cells called cementocytes. Acellular cementum is usually immediately adjacent to the dentin.

Let us briefly summarize the function of cementum:
(1) it anchors the tooth to the alveolus via the periodontal ligament
(2) compensates for tooth wear
(3) contributes to continuous eruption of the teeth. Excessive cementum deposition is called hypercementosis. You will see it on extracted teeth.

COMPARISON OF TISSUES OF THE TEETH

Legend: (E)=Enamel; (D)=Dentin; (C)=Cementum; (P)=Pulp
----
(1)-Mineral Content: (E)=96%; (D)=70%; (C)=50%; (P)=no mineral except denticles or pulpstones.
(2)-Color: (E)=translucent yellow to grayish white; (D)=light yellow; (C)=light yellow; (P) blood red
(3)-Formative Cells: (E)=ameloblast; (D)=odontoblast; (C)=cementoblast; (P) dental papilla
(4)-Embryology: (E)=epithelial; (D)=ectomesenchyme; (C)=ectomesenchyme; (P)=ectomesenchyme
(5)-Repair: (E)=no replacement but sssome remineralization; (D)=physiological, reparative secondary dentin; (C)=new cementum deposition; (P)=can recover from mild inflammation, but severe inflammation results in death

(6)-Aging: (E)=wear, staining, dental caries and physical damage; (D)=increase in secondary and sclerotic dentin; (C)=increased amount with age, more so at the apex; (P)=reduced in size and may be obliterated
(7)-Sensitivity: (E)=none; (D)=yes, only as pain; (C)=no; (P)=yes
(8)-Cells in Mature Tissue: (E)=none; (D)=cytoplasmic extensions from the odontoblasts; (C)=cementocytes are in lacunae; (P)=odontoblasts and other cell types

Investing Structures

A. Periodontal ligament (PDL)
This is the soft specialized connective tissue located between the cementum covering the root of the tooth and the bone forming the alveolus, the bone of the tooth socket. Its average width is approximately 0.2 mm. Its principle function is to support the tooth in its socket. It also has an important function, as you have experienced if you have unexpectedly bitten into something hard. The fibers of the PDL 'suspend' the tooth in its socket; the ends of the fibers attach firmly into the cementum and bone respectively.

Mechanically, the suspension of the tooth is best understood as analogous to a hammock. Orthodontic treatment is possible because the PDL continuously responds and changes as the result of the functional requirements imposed upon it by externally applied forces.

B. Alveolar bone
Anatomically, alveolar bone is the bone of the maxilla and mandible that contains the alveoli for the teeth. It provides support and protection for the teeth. The following concept is important: the alveolar bone is dependent on the functional forces exerted upon the teeth to maintain its structure.

When the teeth are lost, the alveolar bone, in time will be lost also. This alveolar bone presents a special challenge to the dentist when making a denture for geriatric patients who have been edentulous for many years.

C. Oral mucosa
The oral cavity is lined by a mucous membrane whose major functions are lining and protecting. It also serves as a mobile tissue that permits free movement of the lips and cheeks. A unique feature of the oral mucousa is that it is perforated by the teeth. Oral mucosa consists of:
(1) lining mucosa (mobile regions of the oral cavity)
(2) specialized mucosa (the tongue and taste buds)
(3) masticatory mucosa (gingiva and hard palate)

D. Gingiva

This is the specialized mucosa surrounding the erupted teeth. It is arbitrarily divided as follows:

(1) free gingiva, the rolled collar of tissue that surrounds the tooth
(2) attached gingiva, the stippled (like an orange peel) keratinized masticatory mucosa that is firmly bound down to the underlying bone. It is separated from the free gingiva by the free gingival groove (not present in all people) and from the alveolar mucosa by the mucogingival junction. These distinctions are clinically important.

E. Temporomandibular joint
This is the articulation between the mandible and the bilateral temporal bones of the skull. It is a bilateral articulation, that is to say, the right and left sides work as a unit. It is a joint of some complexity that permits hinge motion, protrusion of the mandible, and side-to-side excursion. Put your little fingers into each ear and you can feel the mandibular condyle in motion. You will learn much about the TMJ in your four years in dental school.

F. Saliva and plaque
Saliva is a complex fluid that continuously bathes the teeth. It is produced by three major paired glands (parotid, sublingual, and submandibular) and also by the minor salivary glands. Saliva keeps the mouth moist, helps in mastication and contains a digestive enzyme (amylase). Dental plaque, which we treat as a 'bad guy' is always present. It contains microorganisms, salivary proteins, shed epithelial cells, and the foods we eat. Saliva is very important in dental health. Incidentally, saliva inhibits the HIV virus.

Deciduous Dentition

It is also known as the primary, baby, milk or lacteal dentition.

A. Overview. You will recall that we are diphyodont, that is, with two sets of teeth. The term deciduous means literally 'to fall off.'

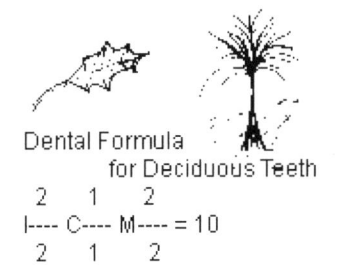

Dental Formula for Deciduous Teeth

$$I\frac{2}{2} \: C\frac{1}{1} \: M\frac{2}{2} = 10$$

There are twenty deciduous teeth that are classified into three classes. Do you recall the term heterodont? There are ten maxillary teeth and ten mandibular teeth. The dentition consists of incisors, canines and molars.
The dental formula is as follows.

$$I\frac{2}{2} \: C\frac{1}{1} \: M\frac{2}{2} = 10$$

-The notation for deciduous teeth is A though J, K through T. It is 'clockwise' just like it is for permanent teeth as you look at the patient from in front.

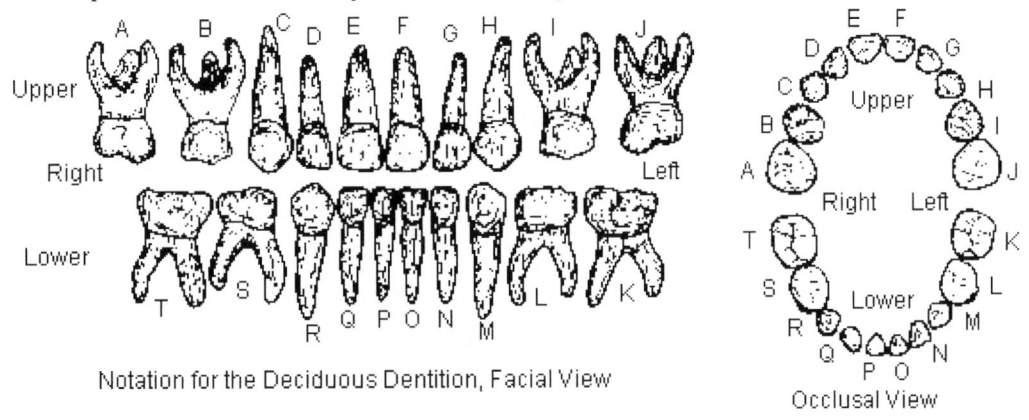

Notation for the Deciduous Dentition, Facial View

Occlusal View

B. Role in development. A person 70 years old will have spent 91% of his/her life chewing on permanent teeth, but only 6% of his/her chewing career with the deciduous dentition.
Although the deciduous teeth are in time replaced by the succedaneous teeth, the deciduous teeth play a very important role in the proper alignment, spacing, and occlusion of the permanent teeth.

The deciduous incisor teeth are functional in the mouth for approximately five years, while the deciduous molars are functional for approximately nine years. They therefore have considerable functional significance. When second deciduous molars are lost prematurely, this can be very detrimental to the alignment of the permanent teeth.

II. Formation and Eruption of Deciduous Teeth.
-Calcification begins during the fourth month of fetal life. By the end of the sixth month, all of the deciduous teeth have begun calcification.
-Clinical hint: good nutrition is essential.

-By the time the deciduous teeth have fully erupted (two to two and one half years of age), cacification of the crowns of permanent teeth is under way. First permanent molars have begun cacification at the time of birth. Clinical hint: with deciduous molars, extract with caution.

Order for Eruption

(deciduous teeth) is as follows:
(1) Central incisor.........Lower 6 ½ months, Upper 7 ½ months
(2) Lateral incisor.........Lower 7 months, Upper 8 months
(3) First deciduous molar...Lower 12-16 months, Upper 12-16 months
(4) Deciduous canine........Lower 16-20 months, Upper 16-20 months
(5) Second deciduous molar..Lower 20-30 months, Upper 20-30 months

Root Formation and Obliteration
A. In general, the root of a deciduous tooth is completely formed in just about one year after eruption of that tooth into the mouth.
B. The intact root of the deciduous tooth is short lived. The roots remain fully formed only for about three years.
C. The intact root then begins to resorb at the apex or to the side of the apex, depending on the position of the developing permanent tooth bud.
D. Anterior permanent teeth tend to form toward the lingual of the deciduous teeth, although the canines can be the exception. Premolar teeth form between the roots of the deciduous molar teeth.

The Transition from the Deciduous to the Permanent Dentition
A. The transition begins with the eruption of the four first permanent molars, and replacement of the lower deciduous central incisors by the permanent lower central incisors.
B. Complete resorption of the deciduous tooth roots permits exfoliation of that tooth and replacement by the permanent (successional) teeth.
C. The mixed dentition exists from approximately age 6 years to approximately age 12 years. In contrast, the intact deciduous dentition is functional from age 2 - 2 /2 years of age to 6 years of age.

D. The enamel organ of each permanent anterior tooth is connected to the oral epithelium via a fibrous cord, the gubernaculum. The foramina through which it passes can be seen in youthful skulls.

Deciduous Dentition

A. It is what the child chews, speaks, and smiles with during his/her formative years. The functional and esthetic importance of these teeth is self evident. The challenge for the clinician lies in communicating with dollar conscious parents who say: "those are just baby teeth. They will just fall out soon."
B. As a rule, these teeth should be restored and preserved until their normal time of exfoliation. This statement especially applies to second molars.
C. The deciduous second molars are particularly important. It is imperative that the deciduous second molars be preserved until their normal time of exfoliation. This prevent mesial migration of the first permanent molars.

Differences Between the Deciduous and Permanent Teeth
A. Deciduous teeth are fewer in number and smaller in size but the deciduous molars are wider mesiodistally than the premolars. The deciduous anteriors are narrower mesiodistally than their permanent successors. Remember the leeway space that we discussed in the unit on occlusion?
B. Their enamel is thinner and whiter in appearance. Side by side, this is obvious in most young patients.
C. The crowns are rounded. The deciduous teeth are constricted at the neck (cervix).
D. The roots of deciduous anterior teeth are longer and narrower than the roots of their permanent successors.
E. The roots of deciduous molars are longer and more slender than the roots of the permanent molars. Also, they flare greatly.
F. The cervical ridges of enamel seen on deciduous teeth are more prominent than on the permanent teeth. This 'bulge' is very pronounced at the mesiobuccal of deciduous first molars.
G. Deciduous cervical enamel rods incline incisally/occlusally.

Deciduous Anterior Teeth
-The primary anteriors are morphologically similar to the permanent anteriors.
-The incisors are relatively simple in their morphology.
-The roots are long and narrow.
-When compared to the permanent incisors, the mesiodistal dimension is relatively larger when compared to axial crown length. In other words, they look 'squatty,' especially when worn.
-At the time of eruption, mamelons are not present in deciduous incisors. (Did you catch that?)
-They are narrower mesiodistally than their permanent successors.

Summary

- Upper molars have three roots, lowers have two roots.
- Upper and lower second deciduous molars resemble first permanent molars in the same quadrant.
- Upper first deciduous molars vaguely resemble upper premolars. -Lower first deciduous molars are odd and unique unto themselves.
- First deciduous molars (upper and lower) have a prominent bulge of enamel on the buccal at the mesial. These help in determining right and left. (Incidentally, there is a somewhat similar bulge of enamel seen on the permanent lower second molar. It is helpful in determining right and left.)

The size of the teeth and the timing of the developing dentition and its eruption are genetically determined. Teeth are highly independent in their development. Also, teeth tend to develop along a genetically predetermined course. One further comment on this issue: tooth development and general physical development are rather independent of one another. Serious illness, nutritional deprivation, and trauma can significantly impact development of the teeth. This genetic independence (and their durability) gives teeth special importance in the study of evolution.

Teeth erupt full size and are ideal for study throughout life. Furthermore, in living people, dental casts and X-ray films are obtained with relative ease. Most important, age and sex can be recorded. With loose teeth in museum collections, age and sex cannot be determined with reliability.

When teeth erupt into the oral cavity, a new set of factors influence tooth position. As the teeth come into function, genetic and environment determine tooth position. For example, tooth arrangement is affected by muscle pressure, as we will discuss shortly.

One final comment: in this course, we treat teeth as a unisex topic. In real life, however, girls shed deciduous teeth and receive their permanent teeth slightly earlier than boys, possibly reflecting the earlier physical maturation achieved by girls. Teeth are slightly larger in boys that in girls; however, we cannot make that distinction by looking at a single extracted tooth.

Occlusion

Occlusion defined: In dentistry, occlusion usually means the contact relationship in function. Concepts of occlusion vary with almost every specialty of dentistry. Here, now, is an introductory definition for one type of occlusion, centric occlusion.

Centric occlusion is the maximum contact and/or intercuspation of the teeth. Comment: this is a static definition--it describes just one position in the chewing cycle.

Occlusion is the sum total of many factors.
1. Genetic factors
Teeth can vary in size. Examples are microdontia (very small teeth) and macrodontia (very large teeth). The shape of individual teeth can vary (such as third molars and the upper lateral incisors.)
They can vary when and where they erupt, or they may not erupt at all (impaction). Teeth can be congenitally missing (partial or complete anodontia), or there can be extra (supernumerary) teeth.
The skeletal support (maxilla/mandible) and how they are related to each other can vary considerably from the norm.

2. Environmental factors
-Habits can have an affect: wear, thumbsucking, pipestem or cigarette holder usage, orthodontic appliances, orthodontic retainers have an influence on the occlusion.

3. Muscular pressure
-Once the teeth erupt into the oral cavity, the position of teeth is affected by other teeth, both in the same dental arch and by teeth in the opposing dental arch.
-Teeth are affected by muscular pressure on the facial side (by cheeks/lips) and on the lingual side (by the tongue).

Occlusion constantly changes with development, maturity, and aging.
1. There is change with the eruption and shedding of teeth as the successional changes from deciduous to permanent dentitions take place.
2. Tooth wear is significant over a lifetime. Abrasion, the wearing away of the occlusal surface reduces crown height and alters occlusal anatomy.
Attrition of the proximal surfaces reduces the mesial-distal dimensions of the teeth and significantly reduces arch length over a lifetime.
3. Tooth loss leaves one or more teeth without an antagonist. Also, teeth drift, tip, and rotate when other teeth in the arch are extracted.

(Stages of dentofacial development)

This presentation is about the development of occlusion. An obvious omission is what happens before birth: that will be covered by others in oral biology. You should know a few things now, however, about events before birth. The very first histological evidence of tooth development appear during the second month of intrauterine life. Calcification of deciduous incisors begins at 3-4 months in utero. By the time of birth, calcification of all the deciduous teeth is well under way.

A. The pre-dentition period
This is from birth to six months.
At this stage, there are no teeth. Clinically, the infant is edentulous (without teeth, remember?).
Both jaws undergo rapid growth; the growth is in three planes of space: downward, forward, and laterally (to the side). Forward growth for the mandible is greater.
The maxillary and mandibular alveolar processes are not well developed at birth. occasionally, there is a neonatal tooth present at birth. It is a supernumerary and is often lost soon after birth.
At birth, bulges in the developing alveoli precede eruption of the deciduous teeth. At birth, the molar pads can touch.
-Comment: When crowns are fully calcified, their growth in size is completed. Therefore, it is a challenge for teeth of a fixed size to accomodate into rapidly growing jaws. One way this challenge is met is by teeth maturing progressively from anterior to posterior in their respective arches.

B. Deciduous dentition period

-The deciduous teeth start to erupt at the age of six months and the deciduous dentition is complete by the age of approximately two and one half years of age.
-The jaws continue to increase in size at all points until about age one year.
-After this, growth of the arches is lengthening of the arches at their posterior (distal) ends. Also, there is slightly more forward growth of the mandible than the maxilla.

1. Many early developmental events take place.
-The tooth buds anticipate the ultimate occlusal pattern.
-Mandibular teeth tend to erupt first. The pattern for the deciduous incisors is usually in this distinctive order:
(1) mandibular central
(2) maxillary central incisors
(3) then all four lateral incisors.

-By one year, the deciduous molars begin to erupt.
-The eruption pattern for the deciduous dentition as a whole is:
(1) central incisor
(2) lateral incisor
(3) deciduous first molar
(4) then the canine
(5) then finally the second molar.
-Remember, we are talking about primary teeth!

-If deciduous teeth are retained too long, consider ankylosed teeth or missing or impacted teeth.
-Eruption times can be variable. If you see a child who is unusually early or late in getting their teeth, inquire about older siblings or parents.

1. Occlusal changes in the deciduous dentition.

The size of the maillary arch tends to be greater than that of the mandibular arch. Therefore, when they are 'superimposed' one atop the other, the maxillary teeth 'overhang' the mandibular teeth

The overjet tends to diminish with age. Wear and mandibular growth are a factor in this process.

The overbite often diminishes with the teeth being worn to a flat plane occlusion.

Often the deciduous teeth are badly chipped and worn. The 'flat plane' occlusion', unusual in our fast food culture was the norm in food forager and early agricultural societies when food contained grit from mill stones.

Spacing of the incisors in anticipation of the soon-to-erupt permanent incisors appears late.

-Primate spaces occur in about 50% of children. They appear in the deciduous dentition. The spaces appear between the upper lateral incisor and the upper canine. They also appear between the lower canine and the deciduous first

C. Mixed Dentition Period.
Begins with the eruption of the first permanent molars distal to the second deciduous molars. These are the first teeth to emerge and they initially articulate in an 'end-on' (one on top of the other) relationship.
-On occasion, the permanent incisors 'spread out' due to spacing. In the older literature, is called by the 'ugly duckling stage.' With the eruption of the permanent canines, the spaces often will close.
-Between ages 6 and 7 years of age there are:
20 deciduous teeth
4 first permanent molars
28 permanent tooth buds in various states of development

1. Errors in development. These are usually genetic.
a. Variability of the individual teeth. In general, the teeth most distal in any class are the most variable.
b. Partial or total anodontia. When yousee missing teeth in children, always ask about the family history. Heredity is significant.
c. Supernumerary teeth.

d. Microdontia
e. Macrodontia
f. Microdontia

2. Errors in skeletal alignment. Malpositioned jaws disrupt normal tooth relationships.

3. Soft tissue problems
-In the mixed dentition, the deciduous second molars have a special importance for the integrity of the permanent dentition. Consider this: The first permanent molars at age six years erupt distal to the second deciduous molars.
-Permanent posterior teeth exhibit physiological mesial drift, the tendency to drift mesially when space is available. If the deciduous second molars are lost prematurely, the first permanent molars drift anteriorly and block out the second premolars. If a second deciduous molar is extracted prematurely, a space maintainer can be fabricated by the dentist.

An incisor diastema may be present. The plural for diastema is diastemata.
-Important: The deciduous anteriors--incisors and canines are narrower than their permanent successors mesiodistally.
-Important: The deciduous molars are wider that their permanent successors mesiodistally.
-This size difference has clinical significance. The difference is called the leeway space.
-The leeway space in the upper arch is approximately 1.8 mm.* In normal development, the leeway space is taken up by the mesial migration of the first permanent molars.

Permanent dentition period

-Maxillary / mandibular occlusal relationships are established when the last of the deciduous teeth are lost. The adult relationship of the first permanent molars is established at this time.

-Occlusal and proximal wear reduces crown height to the permanent dentition and the mesiodistal dimensions of the teeth.

-The proximal wear results in a decrease in arch length. In some persons, the proximal wear per arch can be dramatic. Losses of 1 cm or more have been reported.

-Comment: occlusal and proximal wear also changes the anatomy of teeth. As cusps are worn off, the occlusion can become virtually flat plane. Some speculate that this is the 'normal' condition for an adult occlusion--something we do not see because of soft contemporary diets. Teeth worn to flat plane have exposed dentin, something we consider pathological, but is the normal circumstance amongst many precontact aboriginal peoples. There is a practical advantage to proximal wear: less incisor crowding and fewer impacted third molars. In our culture, we need orthodontic retainers and the skills of oral surgeons.

-In the absence of rapid wear, overbite and overjet tend to remain stable.
-Mesio-distal jaw relationships tend to be stable, except for changes due to disease such as acromegaly (an endocrine disease) or accident.

-Teeth are lasting longer nowadays, thanks to fluoride and advances in dental care.

-With aging, the teeth change in color from off white to yellow. smoking and diet can accelerate staining or darkening of the teeth.

-Gingival recession results in the incidence of more root caries. People are keeping their teeth longer, thus there is more opportunity for root caries

-For most people, teeth become less sensitive cosmetically since the patient to hot and cold, thanks to secondary dentin. With gingival recession, some patients have sensitivity due to exposed dentin at the cemento-enamel junction.

Curve of Spee

-The cusp tips and incisal edges align so that there is a smooth, linear curve when viewed from the lateral aspect. The mandibular curve of Spee is concave whereas the maxillary curve is convex.

-It was described by Von Spee as a 4" cylinder that engages the occlusal surfaces.

-It is called a compensating curve of the dental arch.
-There is another: the Curve of Wilson. Clinically, it relates to the anterior overbite: the deeper the curve, the deeper the overbite. The Curve of Wilson is referred to only infrequently in dental literature.

-If the Curve of Spee is flattened out during orthodontic treatment, it tends to come back.

Overjet and overbite

These are genetic in origin, but can be altered by environment Excessive thumbsucking can increase overjet, for example. In deciduous teeth, they tend to diminish with age. In our culture, they tend to be stable in adults. They diminished in Stone Age man as the teeth were worn to a flat plane. The overwhelming mechanical reason for overjet is that the upper arch is larger and overlies the lower.

Compensating curvatures of the individual teeth.

-This describes the gentle curvature of the long axes of certain posterior teeth to exhibit a gentle curvature.
-These are probably analogous to the trabecular patterns seen in the femur and therefore reflect lines of stress experienced during function.
-Spirals and helices are often encountered in nature. Examples are pubic hair, untrimed finger and toe nails, tusks in elephants, and growing incisors in rodents.

Posteruptive tooth movement. These movements occur after eruption of the teeth into function in the oral cavity. These movements, known collectively as occlusomesial forces are discussed below. It is important for you to learn them and understand them now. In recent literature, the two forces listed below are collectively described as 'occlusomesial' forces. For clarity, we here used the older terms.

A. Continuous tooth eruption is just what the term says: the ongoing eruption of teeth after coming into occlusion. This process compensates for occlusal tooth wear. We mentioned before that cementum thickens in older teeth. Cementum deposition and progressive remodelling of the alveolar bone are the growth processes that provide for continuous

B. Physiological mesial drift describes the tendency of permanent posterior teeth to migrate mesially in the dental arch both before and after they come into occlusion. Clinically, it compensates for proximal tooth wear. -Both continuous tooth eruption and physiological mesial drift are well documented, but the underlying mechanisms are poorly understood. Here are some general observations on physiological mesial drift that will help you in your clinical career.

(1) It describes the tendency of posterior teeth to move anteriorly.
(2) It applies to permanent teeth, not deciduous teeth. (See the remarks at the end of this section on why this is so.)
(3) The further you go distally, the stronger is the tendency for drift.
(4) It compensates for proximal wear.
(5) In younger persons, teeth drift bodily; in older persons, they tip and rotate.
(6) Forces that cause it include occlusal forces, PDL contraction, and soft tissue pressures. There may be other more subtle factors as well.

Normal or 'Ideal' Occlusion

-The ideal molar cusp and buccal relationship as described by Angle (the 'father' of modern orthodontics) is for the mesial cusp of the upper first molar to fit into the buccal groove of the lower first molar.

I. Theories of Tooth Eruption.

The beautiful drawings reproduced below come from a 1941 article by Massler and Schour that discusses the various theories of eruption as they were discussed in 1941 (AJO&OS 27: 552-576). You would think that so basic a process in dentistry would be fully resolved by now. It is not. A definitive article by Marks et al (Anat Rec: 245:374-393) published in 1996 still discusses theories. Briefly look over the drawings frame by frame; they nicely illustrate the eruption of the deciduous tooth, shedding, permanent tooth eruption, and--if lost--the edentulous condition.

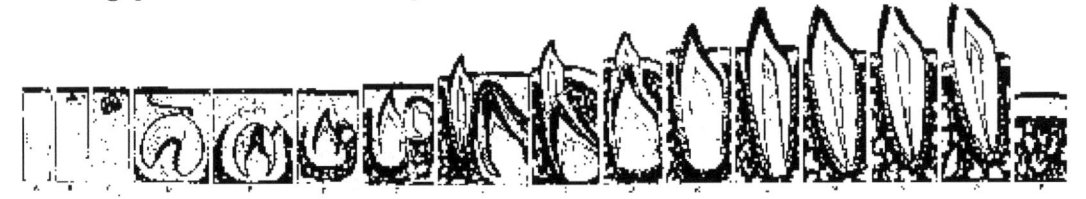

Life History of the Deciduous and Permanent Dentitions, From Massler and Schour, 1941

Tooth eruption is the developmental process whereby the tooth moves in an axial direction from its location within the alveolar crypt of the jaw into a functional position within the oral cavity.

Numerous theories of tooth eruption have been proposed. These theories have involved almost all of the tissues in or near an erupting tooth. None of theories can alone account for all of the movements made by a tooth during its lifetime.

First we will briefly review theories that are NOT ACCEPTABLE.
(1) Vascular pressure and blood vessel thrust. It is well known that the teeth 'jiggle' up and down in synchrony with the arterial pulse. A logical test, therefore is to surgically remove the growing root. When this is done, the tooth continues to erupt. This explanation is not satisfactory.
(2) Pulpal pressure and pulpal growth. Multiplying cells in the root region of the tooth would seem to be an inexorable force in eruption. A test is to excise out the developing tooth, root and all, and replace it with a silicone replica. The result of such a test? The replica erupts as long as the dental follicle is intact. (The dental follicle, also called the dental sac, is the embryonic tissue which goes on to from the cementum, PDL, and the alveolar bone.)

(3) Traction by periodontal fibroblasts. Remember tractor beams in the movie Star Wars? It is that sort of idea. This theory says that fibroblasts tug and pull the developing tooth along its eruptive path. A test of this theory? The administration of drugs that block collage crosslinks have not effect. Teeth continue to erupt without the benefit of fibroblasts.

Next we briefly review some ACCEPTABLE theories.

(1) Root elongation. Root formation would appear to be an obvious cause. Yet, even rootless teeth do erupt. Some teeth will erupt along a greater distance than the length of their completed root.

(2) Alveolar bone remodeling. It is well established that alveolar bone growth, tooth development, and the eruption of the teeth are independent. Bone remodeling in response to orthodontic applicances is an every day occurrence. Also, the alveolar process forms as deciduous teeth erupt and it is lost when teeth are lost as seen most dramatically in older edentulous patients.

(3) Periodontal ligament. In humans, the periodontal ligament DOES NOT seem to be important in eruption. Animal experiments using rats show that the periodontal ligament activity seems important in rodent incisor eruption. This model does NOT apply to humans because rodent incisors grow continuously. Our teeth do not. The only remnant of such growth activity in ourselves are secondary eruption and mesial drift.

In conclusion, it appears that there is no single cause of tooth eruption. Experimental evidence clearly suggest that the dental follicle is an important element in tooth eruption. Study--and debate continue.

II. Butler's Field Theory (Concept of the Morphogenetic Field)
Why are there classes of teeth. In a single person, how do they get that way? Heterodonty, the specialization of teeth into classes has raised a number of theoretical questions. In experimental embryology, the early embryo has been viewed as a mosaic of 'organizational field', each of which pursues its own unique path.
Butler has applied this idea to teeth. It works like this: the tooth row is conceived of as three regions: the incisive region, the canine region, and the molariform. region. Butler includes premolars with molars in the molariform region.

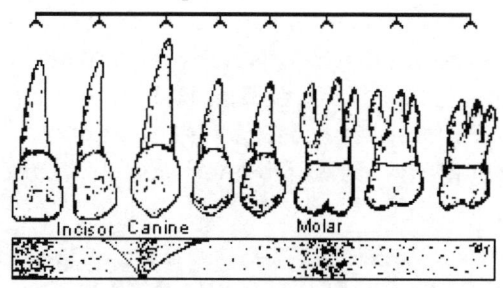

Butler's Concept of the Morphogenetic Field
Presented in a Diagramatic Format
On top is the dental lamina, in the middle the teeth, and in the bottom, field density

In each region, there is a 'best copy', the standard bearer of the group. It is best illustrated with the canine since there is only one in its class. Canines are very stable teeth--and are seldom missing. Lateral incisors are variable in shape (peg-shaped) or are sometimes congenitally missing. In the molariform group, the first permanent molar is the 'best copy' of the group. Second and third upper molars are progressively smaller, the distolingual cusp tends to disappear, and the tooth retreats from being rhomboidal in shape to become a heart shape.

Going anteriorly in the tooth row, the pattern is less clear. Paleontologists tell us that the teeth we know as first and second premolars are actually the third and fourth premolars in the tooth row. Primitive mammals had four premolars. The primitive first and second have been lost. So, in a sense, the premolars most distant from the first permanent molar in the molariform group have been lost altogether. The reaction to the field theory is usually a yawn. Consider it as a springboard for scientific investigation by formulating a hypothesis: Events at one place along the tooth row should have an effect elsewhere along the tooth row. Indeed thisis so. We saw in aprevious unit that when one or more teeth are missing, then there is a greater chance that other teeth will be missing, or at least smaller in size.

The 'field theory' is one of the old war horses in dentistry. If it is applied to experimental work, it can be given new life.

III. Malocclusion, Disuse Theory and the Begg Hypothesis.

Why are so many people wearing 'braces'? Is malocclusion the natural condition for people? Weston Price, a dentist ealier in this century, travelled the world to document the relationship between diet and dental health. His work is ignored today, dismissed for its lack of academic rigor now demanded of scientific literature. The essence of his findings is this: The incidence of malocclusion amongst aboriginal peoples increased after contact with commerercial societies and adoption of a contemporary diet. He found that in precontact aboriginal societies that virtually all individuals show a nearly ideal occlusion. Price attributed malocclusion to a change in diet. Recent evidence suggests that this is only part of the story. Price had attributed malocclusion to nutritional change. He published his definitive work in 1939.

In the 1950s, P. R. Begg, an Australian orthodontist proposed another idea: modern diets prevented the normal wear necessary for a satisfactory occlusion. He studied Australian Aborigine dentitions and observed the considerable occlusal and proximal wear present. Begg concluded that proximal wear on the order of a half inch reduction per arch was normal--and necessary for the occlusion of the teeth. He proposed aggressive action: extraction of teeth to compensate for the lack of proximal wear. We know this theory as the Begg Hypothesis.

Corrucini has gone a step farther with these ideas by returning to one of the oldest theories in orthodontics: the disuse theory. Simply stated, it says that our jaws--particularly the mandible--do not grow to their full potential unless subjected to vigorous use in childhood.

If stated as a proper scientific hypothesis, it is subject to verification or falcification. This is the test of good science. His theory can be stated as follows: Malocclusion results from the lack of chewing stress with modern processed foods. This disuse results in less jaw growth and more malocclusion. In a series of animal experiments with rats and Old World monkeys, Corrucini has confirmed significant dental changes similar to human malocclusion when the test animals are fed soft diets that don't require chewing.

Age and Aging of Teeth

(1) Tooth developmental charts offer many clues, including stages of development for the individual teeth. The neonatal line is a clue to death before birth.
(2) The specific gravity of teeth increases with age.
(3) Individual teeth offer clues as to the age of the individual from whence they came, including clues to age such as blunderbuss root ends, excessive wear, reduced pulp chambers, sclerotic dentin, heavy accretions of dentin.
(4) There is an increase in the hardness with aging.
(5) Tooth wear is increased with age. First permanent molars wear more than seconds; seconds more than thirds.
(6) Sclerotic dentin increases with age. You have seen sclerotic dentin in your laboratory dissections.
(7) The thickness of cernentum increases with age. A very rough rule of thumb is that it doubles in thickness between 25 and 75 years of age.
(8) Teeth tend to darken and acquire stains with age.
(9) Secondary dentin increases with age.

The Permanent Incisor Teeth

Introduction/Morphology/Function/Location

Human incisors have thin, blade-like crowns which are adapted for the cutting and shearing of food. There are two incisors per quadrant, four per arch. The first incisor, the central incisor, is next to the midline. The second incisor, the lateral incisor, is distal to it.

Maxillary incisors by definition arise in the premaxilla (which is merged into the maxilla in humans); mandibular incisors are the teeth that articulate with them.

Maxillary Central Incisor

Facial: It is the most prominent tooth in the mouth. It has a nearly straight incisal edge and a gracefully curved cervical line. The mesial presents a straight outline; the distal aspect is more rounded. Mamelons are present on freshly erupted, unworn central incisors.

Lingual: The lingual aspect presents a distinctive lingual fossa that is bordered by mesial and distal marginal ridges, the incisal edge, and the prominent cingulum at the gingival.

Proximal: Mesial and distal aspects present a distinctive triangular outline. This is true for all of the incisors. The incisal ridge of the crown is aligned on the long axis of the tooth along with the apex of the tooth.
Incisal: The crown is roughly triangular in outline; the incisal edge is nearly a straight line, though slightly crescent shaped.

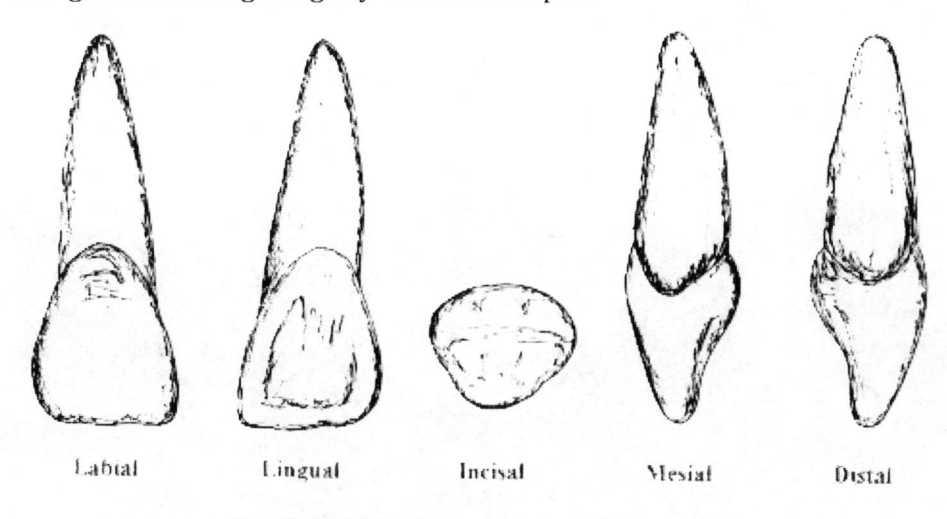

Labial   Lingual   Incisal   Mesial   Distal

Maxillary Right Permanent Central Incisor

Contact Points: The mesial contact point is just about at the incisal, owing to the very sharp mesial incisal angle. The distal contact point is located at the junction of the incisal third and the middle third.

Right and Left: Viewed from the labial, the distal incisal angle is more rounded that the mesial. In many specimens, a cross-section mid-root reveals a right triangle outline. The hypotenuse is toward the mesial.

Variation: The maxillary central incisor usually develops normally. Variations include a short crown or, on occasion, and unusually long crown. This tooth is rarely absent. The Hutchinson incisor is a malformation due to congenital syphilis in utero.

An important non-metric variation of the upper incisors is the shovel shaped incisor trait. It presents with large, robust marginal ridges and a deep lingual fossa. This feature is significant in Chinese, Eskimo-Aleuts, and North American Indians. It is an important clue to population movements, especially those peoples who moved into the Americas from Siberia since the end of the Ice Age.

Maxillary Lateral Incisor

Facial: The maxillary lateral incisor resembles the central incisor, but is narrower mesio-distally. The mesial outline resembles the adjacent central incisor; the distal outline--and particularly the distal incisal angle is more rounded than the mesial incisal angle (which resembles that of the adjacent central incisor. The distal incisal angle resembling the mesial of the adjacent canine.

Lingual: On the lingual surface, the marginal ridges are usually prominent and terminate into a prominent cingulum. There is often a deep pit where the marginal ridges converge gingivally. A developmental groove often extends across the distal of the cingulum onto the root continuing for part or all of its length.

Proximal: In proximal view, the maxillary lateral incisor resembles the central except that the root appears longer--about 1 1/2 times longer than the crown. A line through the long axis of the tooth bisects the crown.

Incisal: In incisal view, this tooth can resemble either the central or the canine to varying degrees. The tooth is narrower mesiodistally than the upper central incisor; however, it is nearly as thick labiolingually.

Labial   Lingual   Incisal   Mesial   Distal

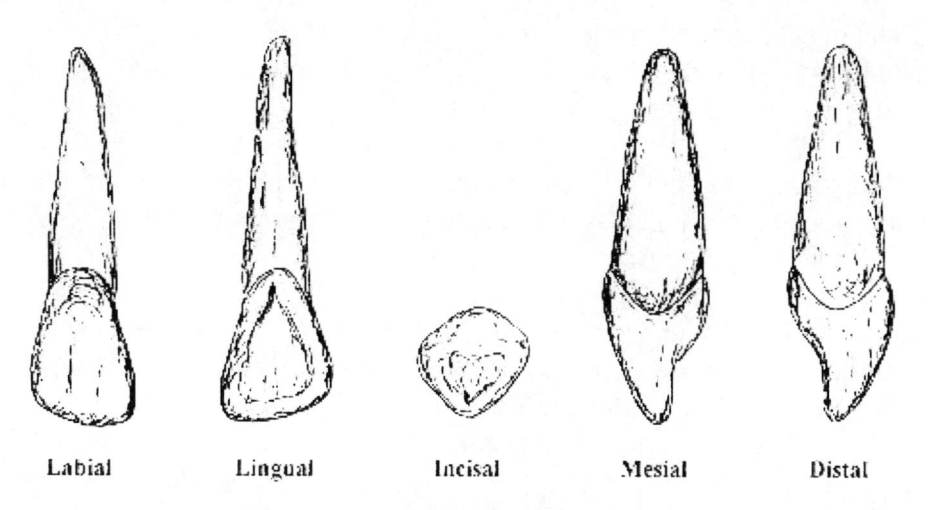

Maxillary Right Permanent Lateral Incisor

Contact Points: The mesial contact is at the junction of the incisal third and the middle third. The distal contact is is located at the center of the middle third of the distal surface.

Right and left: The distoincisal angle is more rounded than the mesial incisal angle. The tip of the root may incline distally, but this is not a consistent finding. Variation: This tooth is quite variable. Often the tooth is narrow, conical, and peg-shaped. It is absent either singly or bilaterally in 1-2% of individuals. Only the lower second premolar is more frequently missing.

The lingual pit when present can be very deep and is prone to early caries in many individuals.

Mandibular Central Incisor

Facial: The mandibular central incisor is the smallest tooth in the dental arch. It is a long, narrow, symmetrical tooth. The incisal edge is straight. Mesial and distal outlines descend apically from the sharp mesial and distal incisal angles.

Lingual: The lingual surface has no definate marginal ridges. The surface is concave and the cingulum is minimal in size.

Proximal: Both mesial land distal surfaces present a triangular outline.

Incisal: The incisal edge is at right angles to a line passing labiolingually through the tooth reflecting its bilateral symmetry.

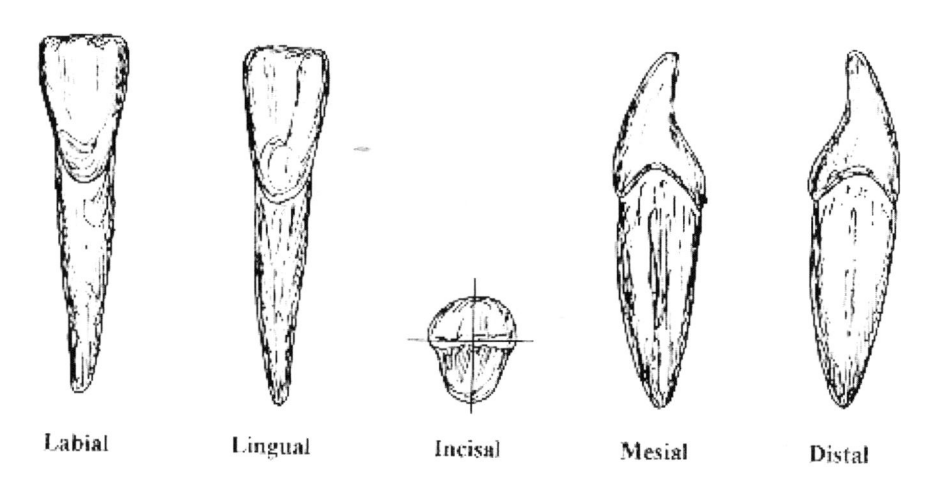

Labial   Lingual   Incisal   Mesial   Distal

Mandibular Right Permanent Central Incisor

Right and Left: The symmetry of this tooth makes a judgement on right and left unreliable.

Variation: This tooth is consistent in development and is is rarely absent. The upper incisor region is a common site for supernumerary teeth which may occasionally occur in the midline; such a variant is called a mesodens.

Mandibular Lateral Incisor

Facial: This tooth resembles the central incisor, but is somewhat larger in most proportions. It is a more rounded tooth; this is especially evident in the distal incisal angle in unworn speciments. There is a lack of the bilateral symmetry seen in the central.

Lingual: Except for the lack of symmetry, this tooth resemble the central.

Proximal: Like the central, the crown presents a triangular outline. When viewed critically, the rotation of the incisal edge can be seen.

Incisal: The incisal edge 'twisted' from the 90 degree angle with a line passing labiolingually through the tooth.

Labial   Lingual   Incisal   Mesial   Distal

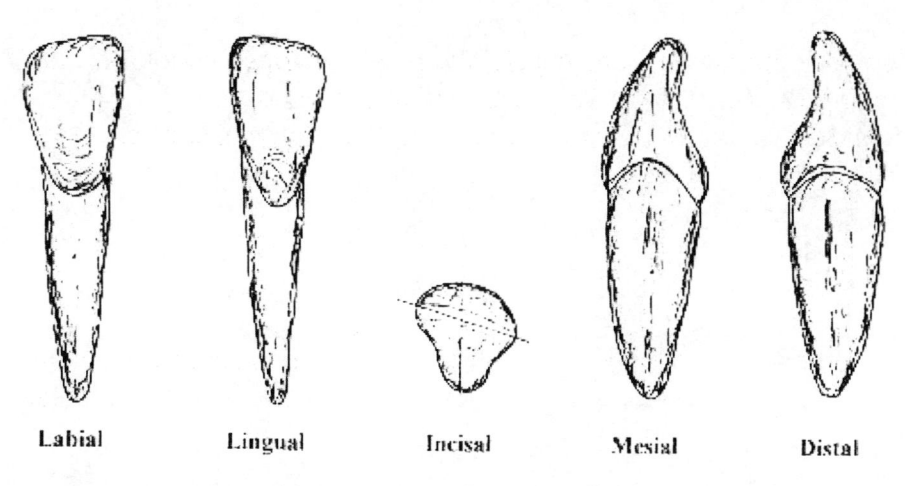

Mandibular Right Permanent Lateral Incisor

Right and Left: Two significant features assist in identification, even in a worn tooth. The incisal edge is 'twisted' relative to a line passing from the labial to the lingual anticipating the curvature of the dental arch. Also, the cingulum will be shifted toward the side from whence the tooth has come.

Variation: This tooth is stable, but variations in root length and direction are occasionally seen.

The Permanent Canine Teeth

Introduction/Morphology/Function/Location

Human canines are the longest and most stable of teeth in the dental arch. Only one tooth of this class is present in each quadrant. In traditional dental literature, canines are considered the cornerstones of the dental arch. They are the only teeth in the dentition with a single cusp. They are especially anchored as prehensile teeth in the group from whence they get their name, the Carnivora.
Maxillary canines by definition are the teeth in the maxilla distal, but closest to the incisors. Mandibular canines are those lower teeth that articulate with the mesial aspect of the upper canine.

Maxillary Permanent Canine

Facial: The canine is approximately 1 mm narrower than the central incisor. Its mesial aspect resembles the adjacent lateral incisor; the distal aspect anticipates the first premolar proximal to it. The canine is slightly darker and more yellow in the color than the incisor teeth. The labial surface is smooth, with a well developed middle lobe extending the full length of the crown cervically from the cusp tip. The distal cusp ridge is longer than the mesial cusp ridge.

Lingual: Distinct mesial and distal marginal ridges, a well-devloped cingulum, and the cusp ridges form the boundries of the lingual surface. The prominent lingual ridge extends from the cusp tip to the cingulum, dividing the lingual surface into mesial and distal fossae.

Proximal: The mesial and distal aspects present a triangular outline. They resemble the incisors, but are more robust--especially in the cingulum region.

Incisal: The asymmetry of this tooth is readily apparent from this aspect. It usually thicker labiolingually than it is mesiodistally. The tip of the cusp is displaced labially and mesial to the central long axis of this tooth.

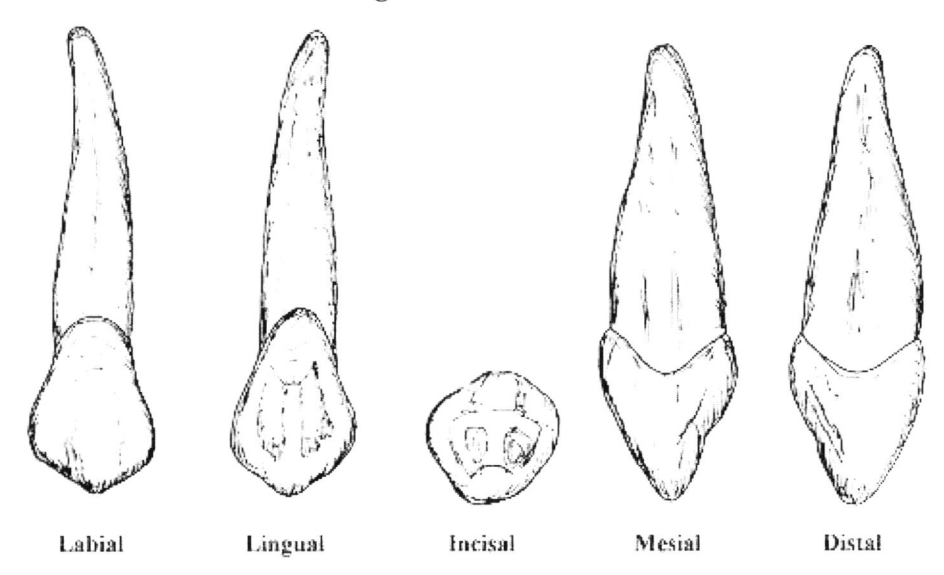

Labial   Lingual   Incisal   Mesial   Distal

Maxillary Right Permanent Canine

Right and Left: The distal surface is fuller and more convex than the mesial surface. The mesial contact point is at the junction of the incisal and middle third. Distally, the contact is situated more cervically. It is at the middle of the middle third.

Variation: Each of the major features of this tooth are 'variations on a theme.' In some persons, a cusp-like tubercle is found on the cingulum. Lingual pits occur only infrequently. On occasion, the root is unusually long or unusually short.

Mandibular Permanent Canine

Facial: The mandibular canine is noticeably narrower mesiodistally than the upper, but the root may be as long as that of the upper canine. In an individual person,the lower canine is often shorter than that of the upper canine. The mandibular canine is wider mesiodistally than either lower incisor. A distinctive feature is the nearly straight outline of the mesial aspect of the crown and root. When the tooth is unworn, the mesial cusp ridge appears as a sort of 'shoulder' on the tooth. The mesial cusp ridge is much shorter than the distal cusp ridge.

Lingual: The marginal ridges and cingulum are less prominent than those of the maxillary canine. The lingual surface is smooth and regular. The lingual ridge, if present, is usually rather subtle in its expression.

Proximal: The mesial and distal aspects present a triangular outline. The cingulum as noted is less well developed. When the crown and root are viewed from the proximal, this tooth uniquely presents a crescent-like profile similar to a cashew nut.

Incisal: The mesiodistal dimension is clearly less than the labiolingual dimension. The mesial and distal 'halves' of the tooth are more identical than the upper canine from this perspective. You will recall that the cusp tip of the maxillary canine is facial to a ling through the long axis. In the mandibular canine, the unworn incisal edge is on the line through the long axis of this tooth.

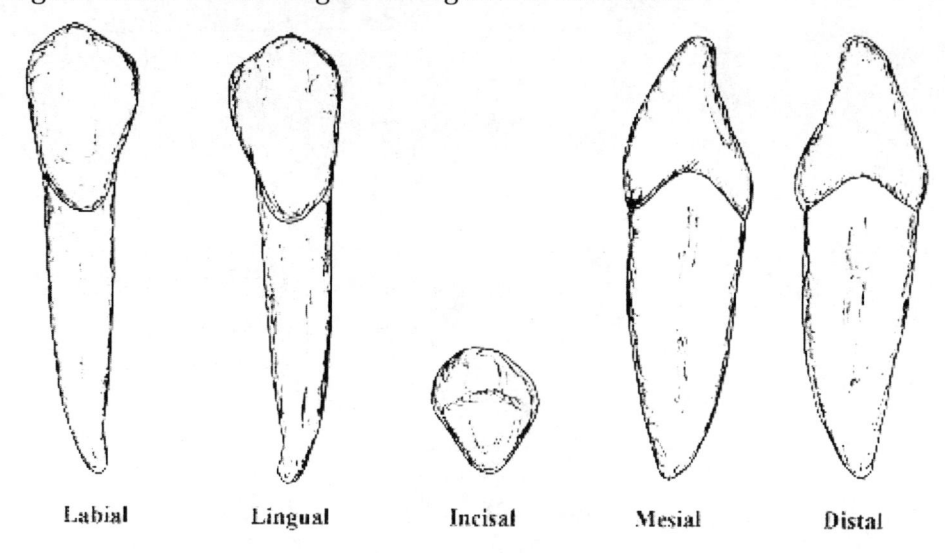

Labial   Lingual   Incisal   Mesial   Distal

Mandibular Right Permanent Canine

Variation: One variation of this tooth has captured the attention of board examiners. It is this: On occasion, the root is bifurcated near its tip. The double root may, or may not be accompanied by deep depressions in the root.

The Premolar Teeth

Introduction/Morphology/Function/Location

The premolar teeth are transitional teeth located between the canine and molar teeth. There are two premolars per quadrant and are identified as first and second premolars. They have at least two cusps. There is always one large buccal cusp, especially so in the mandibular first premolar. The lower second premolar may, at times present with two lingual cusps.

Premolar teeth by definition are permanent teeth distal to the canines preceeded by deciduous molars. In primitive mammals there are four premolars per quadrant.

Maxillary First Premolar

Facial: The buccal surface is quite rounded and this tooth resembles the maxillary canine. The buccal cusp is long; from that cusp tip, the prominent buccal ridge descends to the cervical line of the tooth.

Lingual: The lingual cusp is smaller and the tip of that cusp is shifted toward the mesial. The lingual surface is rounded in all aspects.

Proximal: The mesial aspect of this tooth has a distinctive concavity in the cervical third that extends onto the root. It is called variously the mesial developmental depression, mesial concavity, or the 'canine fossa'--a misleading description since it is on the premolar. The distal aspect of the maxillary first permanent molar also has a developmental depression. The mesial marginal developmental groove is a distinctive feature of this tooth.

Occlusal: There are two well-defined cusps buccal and lingual. The larger cusp is the buccal; its cusp tip is located midway mesiodistally. The lingual cusp tip is shifted mesially. The occlusal outline presents a hexagonal appearance. On the mesial marginal ridge is a distinctive feature, the mesial marginal developmental groove.

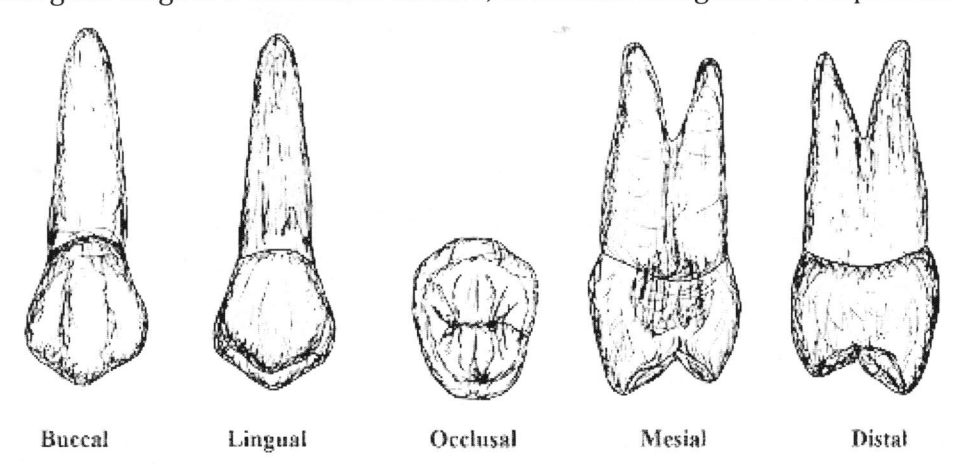

Buccal   Lingual   Occlusal   Mesial   Distal

Maxillary Right First Premolar

Contact Points; Height of Curvature: The distal contact area is located more buccal than is the mesial contact area.

Right and Left: Two distinctive traits help is distinguishing right and left. The mesial developmental depression and the mesially displaced lingual cups tips are consistent clues for determining right and left. When well defined, the mesial marginal ridge is also a clue to right and left.

Root: About 80% of upper premolars have two roots; the next most common variant is a single root.

Variation: Most upper first premolars of people in our society have two roots; however, a single root is found in about 20% of teeth. Three rooted premolars are found occasionally.

Maxillary Second Premolar
Facial: This tooth closely resembles the maxillary first premolar but is a less defined copy of its companion to the mesial. The buccal cusp is shorter, less pointed, and more rounded than the first.

Lingual: Again, this tooth resembles the first. The lingual cusp, however, is more nearly as large as the buccal cusp.

Proximal: Mesial and distal surfaces are rounded. The mesial developmental depression and mesial marginal ridge are not present on the second premolar.

Occlusal: The crown outline is rounded, ovoid, and is less clearly defined than is the first.

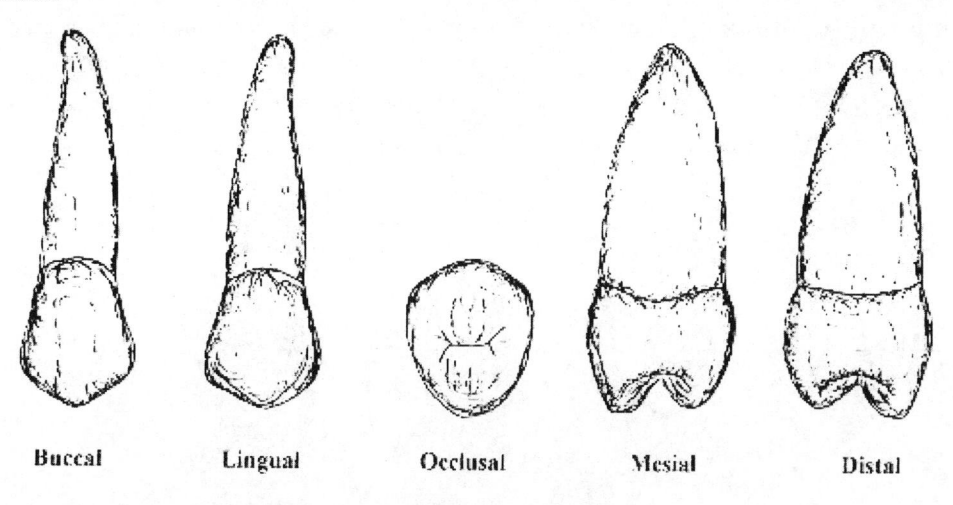

Buccal   Lingual   Occlusal   Mesial   Distal

Maxillary Right Second Premolar

Contact Points; Height of Curvature. When viewed from the facial, the distal contact area is located more cervically than is the mesial contact area.

Right and Left: The one consistent clue to right and left is the lingual cusp tip which is shifted mesially.

Root: The maxillary second premolar has a single root.

Variation: The occlusal anatomy is more variable in the second than in the first. There is wide variability is root size, curvature, and form.

Mandibular First Premolar

Facial: The outline is very nearly symmetrical bilaterally, displaying a large, pointed buccal cusp. From it descends a large, well developed buccal ridge.

Lingual: This tooth has the smallest and most ill-defined lingual cusp of any of the premolars. A distinctive feature is the mesiolingual developmental groove.

Proximal: The large buccal cusp tip is centered over the root tip, about at the long axis of this tooth. The very large buccal cusp and much reduced lingual cusp are very evident. You should keep in mind that the mesial marginal ridge is more cervical than the distal contact ridge; each anticipate the shape of their respective adjacent teeth.

Occlusal: The occlusal outline is diamond-shaped. (Review of premolar occlusal outlines: the upper first is hexagonal, the upper second is ovoid, the lower first is diamond, and the lower second is square.) The large buccal cusp dominates the occlusal surface. Marginal ridges are well developed and the mesiolingual developmental groove is consistently present. There are mesial and distal fossae with pits, affectionately known as 'snake eyes' when they are restored.

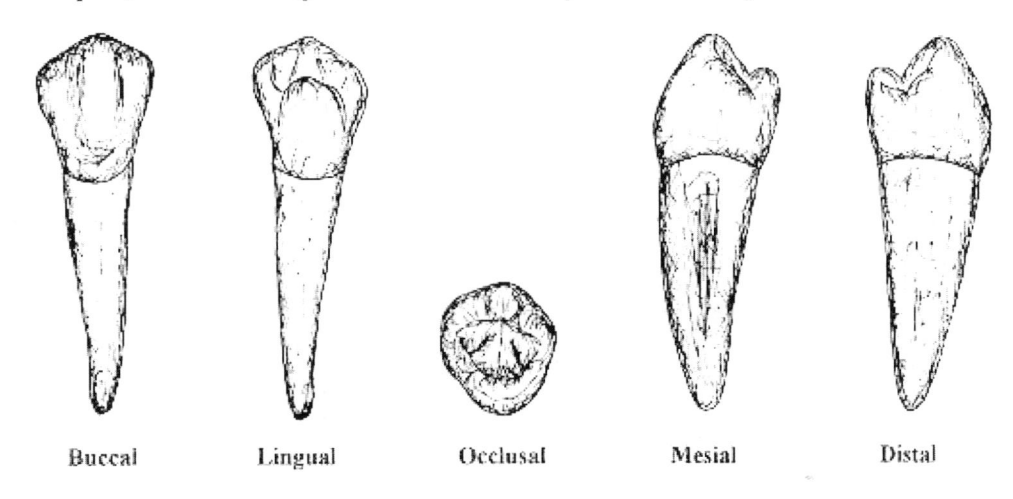

Buccal Lingual Occlusal Mesial Distal

Mandibular Right First Premolar

Contact Points; Height of Curvature: When viewed from the facial, each contact area/height of curvature is at about the same height.

Right and Left: The larger distal occlusal fossa and mesial lingual marginal developmental groove are consistent clues to right and left. The distal surface has a longer radius of curvature than does the mesial surface.

Root: There is a single root. Grooved and/or bifurcated roots do sometimes occur.

Variation: This is a variable tooth in both crown and root. It may, in some persons, more nearly resemble the lower second prmolar.

Mandibular Second Premolar

Facial: From this aspect, the tooth somewhat resembles the first, but the buccal cusp is less pronounced. The tooth is larger than the first.

Lingual: Two significant variations are seen in this view. The most common is the three-cusp form which has two lingual cusps. The mesial of those is the larger of the two. The other form is the two-cusp for with a single lingual cusp. In that variant, the lingual cusp tip is shifted to the mesial.

Proximal: The buccal cusp is shorter than the first. The lingual cusp (or cusps) are much better developed than the first and give the lingual a full, well-developed profile.

Occlusal: The two or three cusp versions become clearly evident. In the three-cusp version, the developmental grooves present a distinctive 'Y' shape and have a central pit. In the two cusp version, a single developmental groove crosses the transverse ridge from mesial to distal.

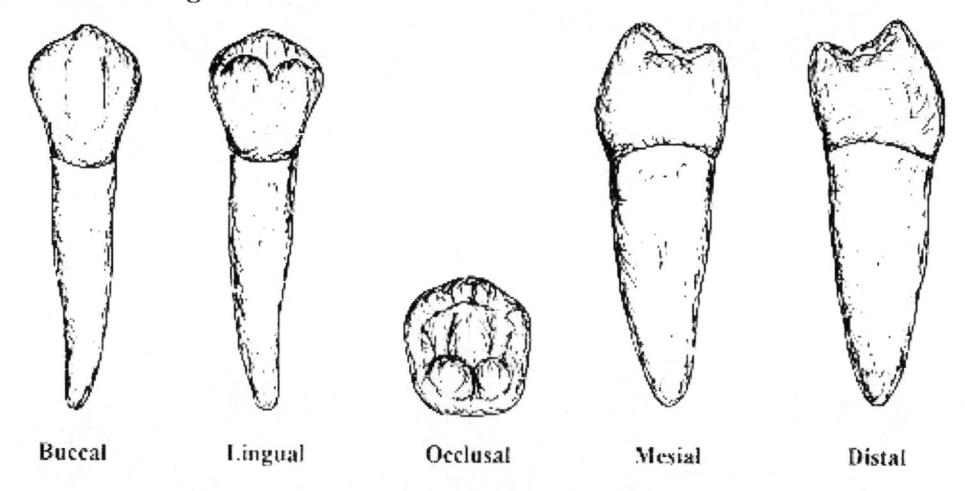

Buccal　　Lingual　　Occlusal　　Mesial　　Distal

Mandibular Right Second Premolar

Contact Points; Height of Curvature: From the facial, the mesial contact is more occlusal than the distal contact. Why? The distal marginal ridge is lower than the mesial marginal ridge.

Right and Left: In the two cusp version, the lingual cusp tip is shifted mesially. In the three cusp version, the larger of the two lingual cusps is to the mesial.

Root: The mandibular second premolar has a single root that is usually larger than that of the first premolar.

Variation: There may be one or two lingual cusps. This tooth is sometimes missing; only the third molars and upper lateral incisors are missing more frequently than this tooth.

The permanent molars occupy the most posterior portion of the dental arch. They have the largest occlusal surfaces of any of the teeth and have from three to five major cusps. Lower permanent molars always have two lingual cusps; upper permanent molars always have two buccal cusps. Lower molars have two roots; upper molars have three roots.

Molar teeth by definition are cheek teeth that are NOT preceded by primary teeth. Permanent molars are accessional teeth without primary predecessors. In contrast to the molars, permanent incisors, canines, and premolars are succedaneous (successional teeth). Primitive mammals had three molars per quadrant. Humans and most primates retain that number. In humans, these teeth are important in chewing and maintaining the vertical dimension.

Maxillary First Permanent Molar
Facial: The mesiobuccal and distobuccal cusps dominate the facial outline. They are separated by the buccal developmental groove. All three roots are visible. The buccal roots present a 'plier handle' appearance with the large lingual root centered between them.

Lingual: Two cusps of unequal size dominate the occlusal profile. The cusps are separated by the lingual developmental groove which is continuous with the distolingual (or distal oblique) groove. The larger mesiolingual cusp often displays the Carabelli trait. It is a variable feature. It appears most often as a cusp of variable size, but is occasionally expressed merely as a pit.

Proximal: In mesial perspective the mesiolingual cusp, mesial marginal ridge, and mesiobuccal cusp comprise the occlusal outline. When present, the Carabelli trait is seen in this view. In its distal aspect, the two distal cusps are clearly seen; however, the distal marginal ridge is somewhat shorter than the mesial one. A small concavity on the distal surface that continues onto the distobuccal root is occasionally described.

Occlusal: The tooth outline is somewhat rhomboidal with four distinct cusps. The cusp order according to size is: mesiolingual, mesiobuccal, distobuccal, and distolingual. The tips of the mesiolingual, mesiobuccal, and distobuccal cusps form the trigon, reflecting the evolutionary origins of the maxillary molar. The distolingual cusp is called the talon (heel) and is a more recent acquisition in evolutionary history. A frequent feature of maxillary molars is the Carabelli trait located on the mesiolingual cusp.

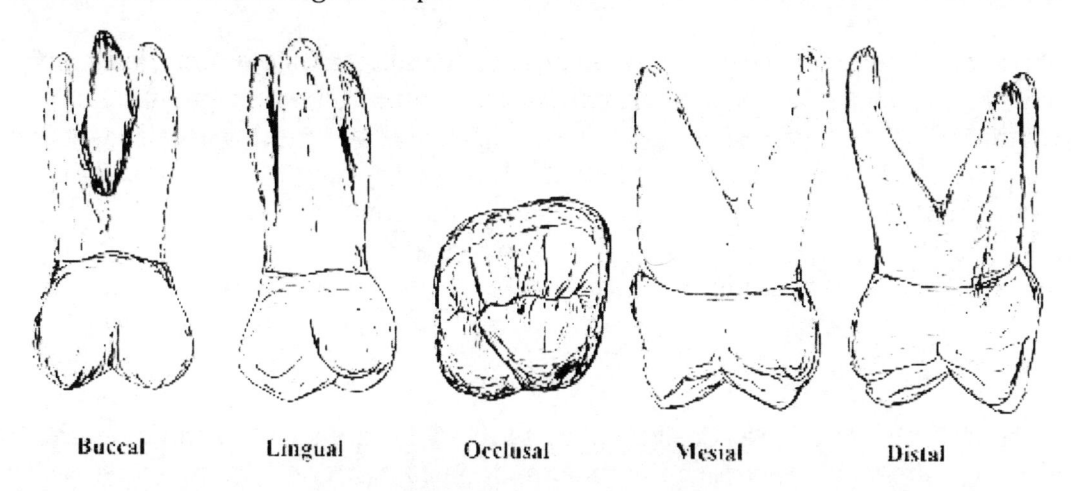

Buccal　　Lingual　　Occlusal　　Mesial　　Distal

Maxillary Right First Permanent Molar

Contact Points; Height of Curvature: The mesial contact is above, but close to, the mesial marginal ridge. It is somewhat buccal to the center of the crown mesiodistally. The distal contact is similarly above the distal marginal ridge but is centered buccolingually.

Right and Left: The large mesiolingual cusp, single large lingual (palatal) root, and Carabelli trait make distinguishing right and left easy.

Roots: There are three roots, two buccal and one lingual. The lingual root is the longest and is often described as 'banana shaped.' The mesiobuccal root is not as long; the distobuccal is the smallest of the three. Observe that the sequence of diminishing root size corresponds to the sequence of diminishing cusp size described above.

Variation: Deviation from the accepted normal is infrequent. The Carabelli trait is a variable feature. It is of special interest to the dental anthropologist in tracing human evolutionary history.

Maxillary Second Permanent Molar
Facial: The crown is shorter occluso-cervically and narrower mesiodistally whe compared to the first molar. The distobuccal cusp is visibly smaller than the mesiobuccal cusp. The two buccal roots are more nearly parallel. The roots are more parallel; the apex of the mesial root is on line with the with the buccal developmental groove. Mesial and distal roots tend to be about the same length.

Lingual: The distolingual cusp is smaller than the mesiolingual cusp. The Carabelli trait is absent.

Proximal: The crown is shorter than the first molar and the palatal root has less diverence. The roots tend to remain within the crown profile.

Occlusal: The distolingual cusp is smaller on the second than on the first molar. When it is much reduced in size, the crown outline is described as 'heart-shaped.' The Carabelli trait is usually absent. The order of cusp size, largest to smallest, is the same as the first but is more exaggerated: mesiolingual, mesiobuccal, distobuccal, and distolingual.

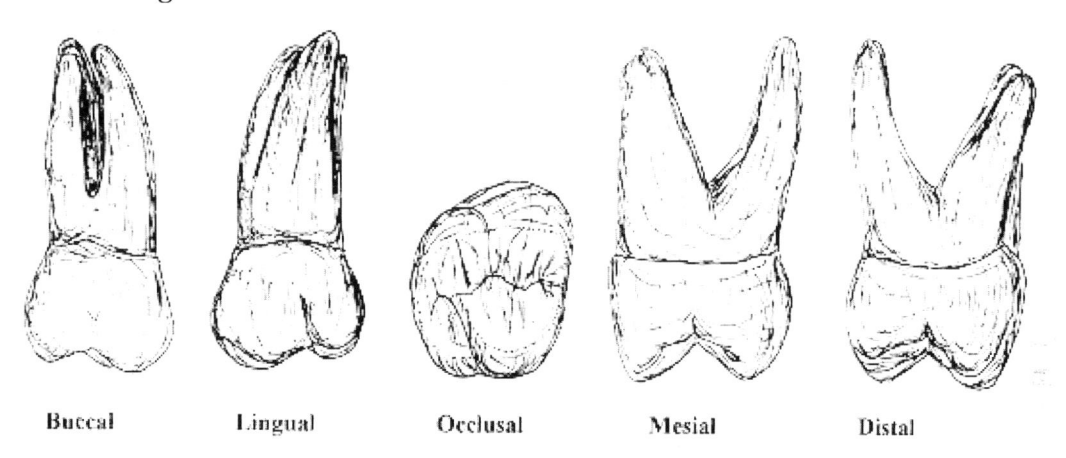

Buccal   Lingual   Occlusal   Mesial   Distal

Maxillary Right Second Permanent Molar

Contact Points; Height of Curvature: Both mesial and distal contacts tend to be centered buccolingually below the marginal ridges. Since themolars become shorter, moving from first to this molar, the contacts tend to appear more toward the center of the proximal surfaces.

Right and Left: The large mesiolingual cusp, small distolingual cusp, and the three roots make distinguishing right and left easy.

Roots: There are three roots, two buccal and one lingual. The roots are less divergent than the first with their apices usually falling within the crown profile. The buccal roots tend to incline to the distal.

Variation: The distolingual cusp is the most variable feature of this tooth. When it is large, the occlusal is somewhat rhomboidal; when reduced in size the crown is described as triangual or 'heart-shaped.' At times, the root may be fused.

Maxillary Third Permanent Molar
Special Note: Maxillary and mandibular third molars show more developmental variation that any of the other permanent teeth. They are the teeth most often congenitally missing.
Facial: The crown is usually shorter in both axial and mesiodistal dimensions. Two buccal roots are present, but in most cases they are fused. The mesial buccal cusp is larger than the distal buccal cusp.

Lingual: In most thirds, there is just one large lingual cusp. In some cases there is a poorly developed distolingual cusp and a lingual groove. The lingual root is often fused to the to buccal cusps.

Proximal: The outline of the crown is rounded; it is often described as bulbous in dental literature. Technically, the mesial surface is the only 'proximal' surface. The distal surface does not contact another tooth.

Occlusal: The crown of this tooth is the smallest of the maxillary molars. The first molar is the largest in the series. The outline of the occlusal surface can be described as heart-shaped. The mesial lingual cusp is the largest, the mesial buccal is second in size, and the distal buccal cusp is the smallest.

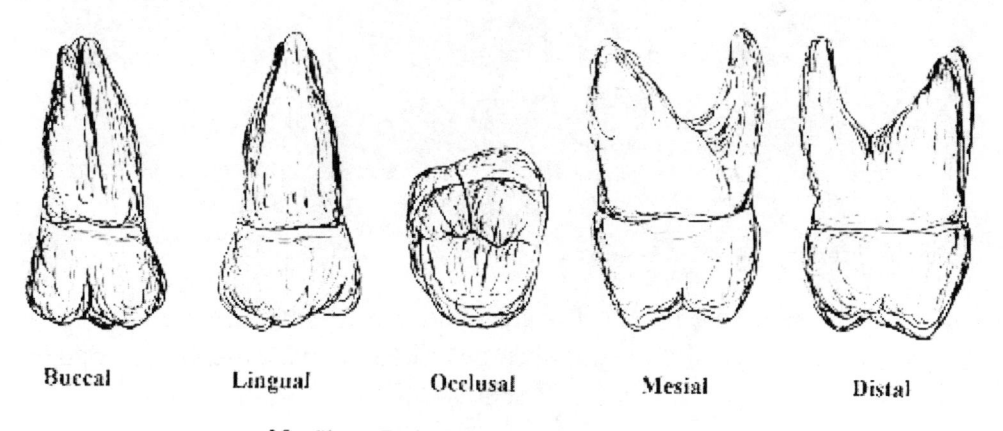

Buccal Lingual Occlusal Mesial Distal
Maxillary Right Third Molar

Contact Points; Height of Curvature: This tooth is rounded and variable in shape. The distal surface has no contact with any other tooth.

Right and Left: Although this tooth is a variable and anomalous tooth, right and left is fairly easy to determine. The mesiobuccal cusp is much larger than the distobuccal cusp. This helps in the determination of right and left.

Roots: There are three roots, two buccal and one lingual; however, they are usually fused into one functional root.

Variation: They are the most variable teeth in the dentition. Impaction occurs frequently. Some resemble the adjacent second molar; others may have many cusps, small 'cusplets', and many grooves.

Mandibular First Permanent Molar
Facial: The lower first permanent molar has the widest mesiodistal diameter of all of the molar teeth. Three cusps cusps separated by developmental grooves make on the occlusal outline seen in this view. Moving from mesial to distal, these features

form the occlusal outline as follows: mesiobuccal cusp, mesiobuccal developmental groove, distobuccal cusp, distobuccal developmental groove, and the distal cusp. The mesiobuccal cusp is usually the widest of the cusps. The mesiobuccal cusp is generally considered the largest of the five cusps. The distal cusp is smaller than any of the buccal cusps and it contributes little to the buccal surface. The two roots of this tooth are clearly seen. The distal root is usually less curved than the mesial root.

Lingual: Three cusps make up the occlusal profile in this view: the mesiolingual, the distolingual, and the distal cusp which is somewhat lower in profile. The mesiobuccal cusp is usually the widest and highest of the three. A short lingual developmental groove separates the two lingual cusps

Proximal: The distinctive height of curvature seen in the cervical third of the buccal surface is called the cervical ridge. The mesial surface may be flat or concave in its cervical third. It is highly convex in its middle and occlusal thirds. The occlusal profile is marked by the mesiobuccal cusp, mesiolingual cusp, and the mesial marginal ridge that connects them. The mesial root is the broadest buccolingually of any of the lower molar roots. The distal surface of the crown is narrower buccolingually than the mesial surface. Three cusps are seen from the distal aspect: the distobuccal cusp, the distal cusp, and the distolingual cusp.

Occlusal: This tooth presents a pentagonal 'home plate' occlusal outline that is distinctive for this tooth. There are five cusps. Of them, the mesiobuccal cusp is the largest, the distal cusp is the smallest. The two buccal grooves and the single lingual groove form the "Y5" patern distinctive for this tooth. The five cusp and "Y5" pattern is important in dental anthropology.

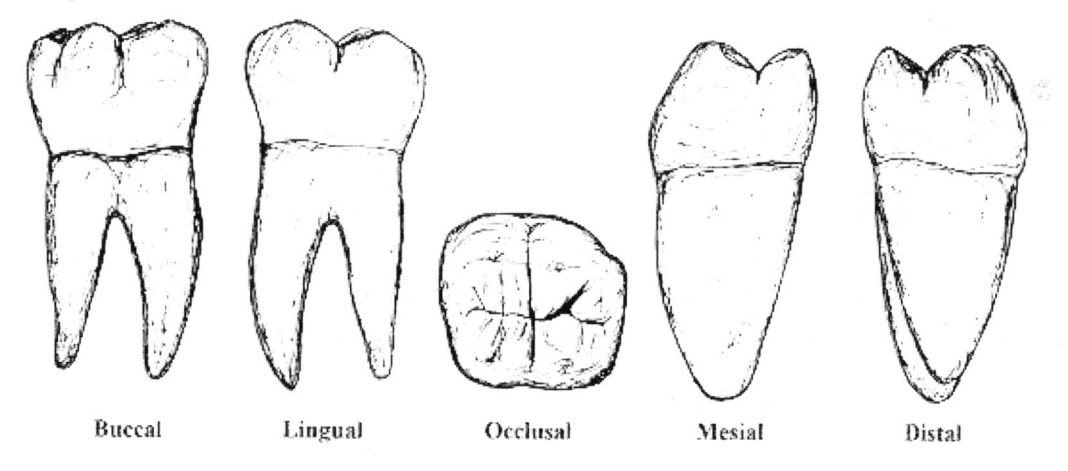

Buccal　　Lingual　　Occlusal　　Mesial　　Distal

Mandibular Right First Permanent Molar

Contact Points; Height of Curvature: The mesial contact is centered buccolingually just below the marginal ridge. The distal contact is centered over the distal root, but is buccal to the center point of the distal marginal ridge.

Right and Left: The cervical ridge on the buccal aspect, the two buccal cusps located to the buccal along with the distal cusp provide identification of the buccal aspect.

The distal cusp is the smallest and is displaced along the occlusal aspect. These features make possible identification of right and left.

Roots: Lower molars have mesial and distal roots. In the first, molar, the mesial root is the largest. It has a distal curvature. The distal root has little curvature and projects distally.

Variation: Most lower first molars have five cusps. Occasionally the distal cusp is missing. More rarely, in large molars, the distal cusp is joined by a sixth cusp, the 'cusp six' or tuberculum sextum

Mandibular Second Molar

Facial: When compared to the first molar, the second molar crown is shorter both mesiodistally and from the cervix to the occlusal surface. The two well-developed buccal cusps form the occlusal outline. There is no distal cusp as on the first molar. A buccal developmental groove appears between the buccal cusps and passes midway down the buccal surface toward the cervix.

Lingual: The crown is shorter than that of the first molar. The occlusal outline is formed by the mesiolingual and distolingal cusps.

Proximal: The mesial profile resembles that of the first molar. The distal profile is formed by the distobuccal cusp, distal marginal ridge, and the distolingual cusp. Unlike the first molar, there is no distal fifth cusp.

Occlusal: There are four well developed cusps with developmental grooves that meet at a right angle to form the distinctive "+4" pattern characteristic of this tooth.

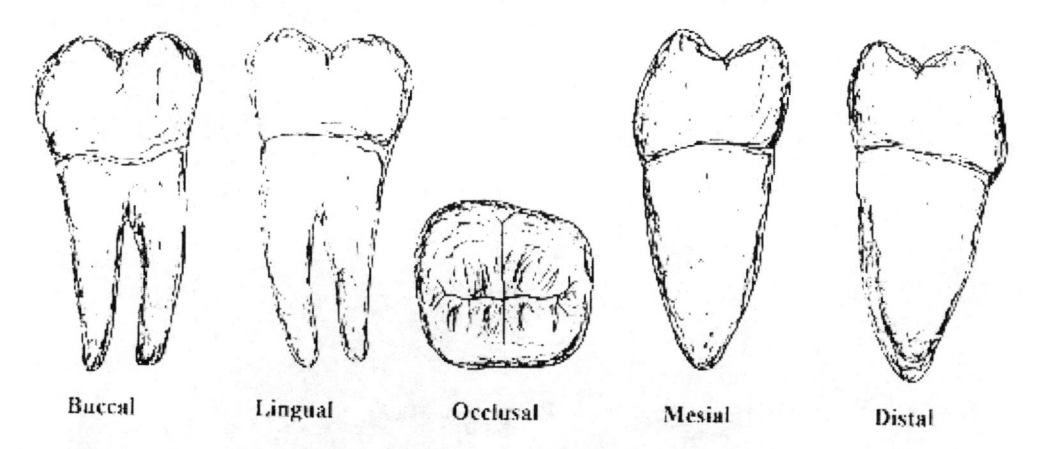

Buccal   Lingual   Occlusal   Mesial   Distal

Mandibular Right Second Permanent Molar

Contact Points; Height of Curvature: When moving distally from first to third molar, the proximal surfaces become progressively more rounded. The net effect is to displace the contact area cervically and away from the crest of the marginal ridges.

Right and Left: When viewed occlusally, there is a distinctive prominence of enamel at the mesiobuccal--a feature shared with first deciduous molars.

Examined from the mesial or distal, the lingual surface has its height of curvature midway between the occlusal and the cervical line. On the buccal surface, the height of curvature is at the gingival third--near the cervical line.

Roots: There are two roots which are often shorter than those of the first. When compared to first molar roots, those of the second tend to be more parallel and to have a more distal inclination.

Variation: Morphologically this is a stable tooth. Five-cusp versions are seen on occasion, however root variability is greater than in the first molar.

Mandibular Third Molar

Facial: The crown is often short and has a rounded outline.

Lingual: Similarly, the crown is short and the crown is bulbous.

Proximal: Mesially and distally, this tooth resembles the first and second molars. The crown of the third molar, however, is shorter than either of the other molars. Technically, only the mesial surface is a 'proximal' surface.

Occlusal: Four or five cusps may be present. This surface can be a good copy of the first or second molar, or poorly developed with many accessory grooves. The occlusal outline is often ovoid and the occlusal surface is constricted. Occasionally, the surface has so many grooves that it is described as crenulated--a condition seen in the great apes.

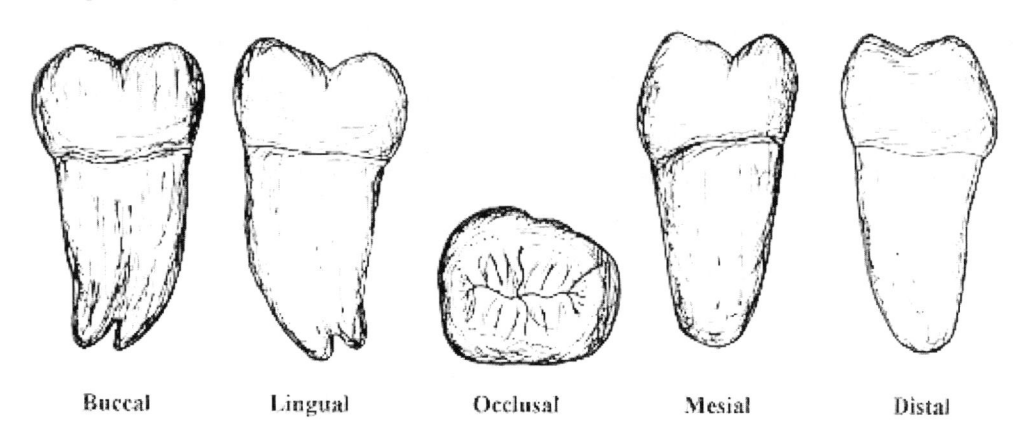

Buccal   Lingual   Occlusal   Mesial   Distal

Mandibular Right Third Molar

Contact Points; Height of Curvature: The rounded mesial surface has its contact area more cervical than any other lower molar. There is no tooth distal to the third molar.

Right and Left: In the five cusp version the buccal side of the tooth is easily identified. This can be confirmed by comparison with the lingual and buccal surface contours. In four cusp versions the mesial cusps are usually more developed than the distal cusps, contributing to this tooth's ovoid occlusal profile.

Roots: The two roots are usually short, often curved distally, and poorly developed.

Variation: This is an extremely variable tooth and on occasion it is missing. While the most common anomalie of upper third molars is that they are undersized, lower third molars can be undersized or oversized. Lower third molars fail to erupt in many persons.

Caries

Caries is the decay process which takes place on a tooth surface. Three criteria are necessary in order to allow for caries development:
Tooth Surface
Bacteria, which metabolize the substrate. The main organisms responsible for this decay are Streptococcus mutans and Lactobacillus
Substrate (i.e. food, sugar)
It is when bacteria metabolize substrate on the tooth surface that caries develop. Therefore, all three of the above must be present together for caries to form. Once caries progress, they eventually form a hole, or cavity, in the tooth. When a cavity is detected, a filling is then placed. If a cavity is not detected, the decay or caries may be small enough that more conservative treatment can be done (see

Stage I of caries classification)
Smooth Surface Caries
This type of decay (triangle-shaped) usually occurs in between teeth, right under the tooth contact, leaving a broad area of decay. In this case, the broad area of decay (base of triangle) is on the surface side of enamel, while the narrow end is towards the dentin (at the dentino-enamel junction - DEJ). As soon as decay hits the DEJ, it spreads laterally along this border.

Fissure Caries
This type of decay (diamond-shaped) usually occurs in deep fissures/grooves on top of the surface of the tooth. Therefore, the narrow end or apex of the triangle points to the surface side of enamel, while the broad base of decay extends towards the DEJ. As soon as decay hits the dentin, it spreads laterally along the DEJ.

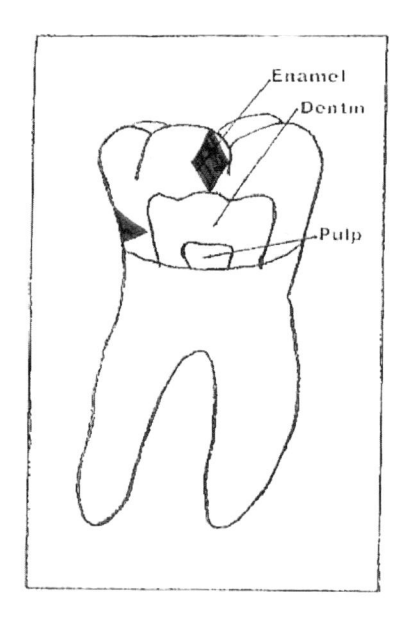

In summary, for both smooth surface and fissure caries, in the dentin, both of these types of caries display a similar triangular pattern of decay, where the broad area of decay is at the DEJ (towards the enamel) and the narrow area of decay (apex) points toward the pulp. However, the pattern of decay in enamel differs between them.

Stage I
As seen in the figure, the decay (triangle) is ALL in enamel and less than half way from the tooth surface to dentin. These are so small that the inserted fillings are either extremely small, or no fillings are opted to be placed at all. In the latter case, fluoride is initiated in the hopes of arresting and potentially reversing the decay process (therefore, at this stage, there is a chance that the enamel can remineralize, thereby eliminating the decay/caries).

Stage II
The decay (triangle) is still ALL in enamel (like stage I), but has passed the half way mark from the tooth surface to the dentin (DEJ). These fillings are still classified as small and may remain within the enamel. However, usually fillings here will extend into the dentin to allow for more retention of the filling.

Stage III
The decay (triangle) has passed the DEJ so it has penetrated ALL of the enamel and has entered into dentin. However, the decay has NOT passed the half-way mark between the DEJ and the pulp (ie. where the dentin began and enamel ended and

where the pulp is).

Stage IV
The decay (triangle) is like stage III, but the decay in dentin has passed the half-way mark from the enamel (DEJ) to the pulp. These fillings will be quite large and if delayed, the decay will spread until it reaches the pulp. This is cause for concern, seeing that the pulp contains vital components such as blood vessels and nerves. Once decay reaches the pulp, a simple filling will no longer suffice and a root canal is needed.

Root Canal
Aside from Stage IV caries, other causes which cause root canals include:
- Root resorption caused by trauma, orthodontic treatment, ectopic eruption, etc.
- Developmental anomalies, such as dens invaginatus
- Propholactically for over dentures, crowns or extreme bruxers, etc

With a root canal, a hole is drilled in the tooth and the pulp is removed. The area where the pulp was removed is then filled and then a permanent filling is placed on top.

Fillings vs. Pit and Fissure Sealants vs. PRR
Fillings- Decay is removed and the hole which was drilled (preparation) is made retentive. This is performed by smooth walls, etc. Following this, a filling is placed inside. The filling is then carved to try to reproduce the anatomy of the tooth. It is important to note that fillings are placed on any tooth in the mouth (not just the molars), and on any surface.

Pit and fissure sealants are a preventative measure (ie, they are done before any actually caries or decay are detected). They are placed in the hopes of preventing the formation of decay and the potential future need for a filling. Sealants and preventative resins are placed only on molars, and on the occlusal / top surfaces of the tooth, while fillings can be placed on any teeth, and on any surface. Therefore, if one sees deep or stained grooves / fissures on the occlusal surface of molars (ie. places where decay has a chance of developing), a sealant is placed to obliterate these grooves.

PRR's (preventative resins) go much much deeper into the tooth (usually into the dentin layer) and are considered less conservative (ie. more tooth structure must be removed because all the decayed tooth must be removed before placing the filling). Placed only on the occlusal surface of molars

Therefore, a tooth with a large amount of decay (ie. extending into the dentin) is treated with a filling, a tooth with an extremely small amount of caries (ie. stage I, where the decay is still in the enamel) is treated with a preventative resin (PRR). Lastly, a tooth with no caries, but has deep or stained grooves and fulfills other indications for a sealants is treated with a pit and fissure sealant, which will prevent the need for a filling or PRR in the future.

Sealants

Sealants are a safe and effective hard material which is placed in the grooves on a tooth surface. They obliterate the grooves, deep pits, fossa and fissures on the upper (occlusal) surface of the molars (the upper portion of the molars where the food gets chewed).

They work in two ways to prevent caries development:
Keeps substrate (i.e. food and bacteria) out of deep pits, grooves and fissures on the teeth.
Create an anaerobic environment which eliminate the aerobic bacteria and other decaying matter residing in this area of the tooth. In cases where a little decay may have been left in deep grooves, cavities may be prevented from spreading since the bacteria are unable to thrive.
Criteria for Sealant Placement:
Generally, there are two criteria used to determine whether or not a patient is a suitable candidate for a sealant placement, namely:
- Deep occlusal fissures present in a carious tooth
- Deep occlusal fossa present in a carious tooth

Indications for sealants:
Antimere (tooth on the opposite side of the mouth) with similar morphology (ie, similar deep groove pattern) has caries/decay or a filling. This is an indication because the tooth on the other side, since it looks the same, represents a similar risk. Therefore, if there is decay or a filling on the antimere tooth, there is a risk that the tooth will decay and later need a filling.

Occlusal restorations (fillings on the tops of the teeth) are needed or are placed on adjacent molars. This is an indication because if the teeth beside the tooth in question have fillings or need fillings, there is a risk of that tooth developing decay.

Shortly following tooth eruption (usually within 3 yrs). This is an indication because within the first 3 years that the tooth has been in the mouth, there is the highest risk of forming decay. Also, if a sealant is to be placed, it needs to be erupted enough so the entire top / occlusal surface of the tooth must be exposed. If this is not the case, one cannot access the surface to place the sealant.

Absence of proximal caries (decay between teeth). This is an indication because if a filling needs to be placed for this type of decay after a sealant has been placed, the sealant will break off.

In conjunction with a fluoride program. This is an indication because fluoride helps reduce the risk of decay and will compliment the role of the sealant in preventing cavities.

Contra-indications for sealants:
Rampant caries / decay. This is a contraindication because in cases where there is so much decay, there will most likely be the need for fillings (i.e. less conservative treatment).

Interproximal lesions (decay between teeth). This is a contraindication because sealants are only placed on the occlusal surface of teeth, and a filling, not a sealant, is needed in between the teeth.

Occlusal surface is already carious (top surface already has decay). This is a contraindication because a sealant will not remove all the decay (it will only remove all of the decay if the amount if extremely small). Instead, a filling is needed.

Dental Emergencies and Treatment

Diagnosis	Definition	Presentation	Complications	Treatment
Reversible pulpitis	Pulpal inflammation	Pain with hot, cold, or sweet stimuli	Periapical abscess, cellulitis	Filling
Irreversible pulpitis	Pulpal inflammation	Spontaneous, poorly localized pain	Periapical abscess, cellulitis	RCT, extraction
Abscess	Localized bacterial infection	Localized pain and swelling	Cellulitis	I & D and RCT or extraction
Cellulitis	Diffuse soft tissue bacterial infection	Pain, erythema, and swelling	Regional spread	Antibiotics and RCT or extraction
Pericoronitis	Inflamed gum over partially erupted tooth	Pain, erythema, and swelling	Cellulitis	Irrigation, antibiotics if cellulitis also present
Tooth fracture	Broken tooth	Clinical examination and radiography	Pulpitis and sequelae	Fillings, with or without RCT, extraction
Tooth luxation	Loose tooth	Clinical examination and radiography	Aspiration, pulpitis, and sequelae	Splinting, with or without RCT, extraction
Tooth avulsion	Missing tooth	Clinical examination	Ankylosis, resorption	Reimplantation and splinting

RCT = root canal therapy; I & D = incision and drainage.

Ellis Classification of Tooth Fractures
I- Enamel only
II- Into the dentin
III- Into the pulp

Secret Key #1 - Time is Your Greatest Enemy

Pace Yourself

Wear a watch. At the beginning of the test, check the time (or start a chronometer on your watch to count the minutes), and check the time after every few questions to make sure you are "on schedule."

If you are forced to speed up, do it efficiently. Usually one or more answer choices can be eliminated without too much difficulty. Above all, don't panic. Don't speed up and just begin guessing at random choices. By pacing yourself, and continually monitoring your progress against your watch, you will always know exactly how far ahead or behind you are with your available time. If you find that you are one minute behind on the test, don't skip one question without spending any time on it, just to catch back up. Take 15 fewer seconds on the next four questions, and after four questions you'll have caught back up. Once you catch back up, you can continue working each problem at your normal pace.

Furthermore, don't dwell on the problems that you were rushed on. If a problem was taking up too much time and you made a hurried guess, it must be difficult. The difficult questions are the ones you are most likely to miss anyway, so it isn't a big loss. It is better to end with more time than you need than to run out of time.

Lastly, sometimes it is beneficial to slow down if you are constantly getting ahead of time. You are always more likely to catch a careless mistake by working more slowly than quickly, and among very high-scoring test takers (those who are likely to have lots of time left over), careless errors affect the score more than mastery of material.

Secret Key #2 - Guessing is not Guesswork

You probably know that guessing is a good idea - unlike other standardized tests, there is no penalty for getting a wrong answer. Even if you have no idea about a question, you still have a 20-25% chance of getting it right.

Most test takers do not understand the impact that proper guessing can have on their score. Unless you score extremely high, guessing will significantly contribute to your final score.

Monkeys Take the Test

What most test takers don't realize is that to insure that 20-25% chance, you have to guess randomly. If you put 20 monkeys in a room to take this test, assuming they answered once per question and behaved themselves, on average they would get 20-25% of the questions correct. Put 20 test takers in the room, and the average will be much lower among guessed questions. Why?

1. The test writers intentionally writes deceptive answer choices that "look" right. A test taker has no idea about a question, so picks the "best looking" answer, which is often wrong. The monkey has no idea what looks good and what doesn't, so will consistently be lucky about 20-25% of the time.
2. Test takers will eliminate answer choices from the guessing pool based on a hunch or intuition. Simple but correct answers often get excluded, leaving a 0% chance of being correct. The monkey has no clue, and often gets lucky with the best choice.

This is why the process of elimination endorsed by most test courses is flawed and detrimental to your performance- test takers don't guess, they make an ignorant stab in the dark that is usually worse than random.

$5 Challenge

Let me introduce one of the most valuable ideas of this course- the $5 challenge:

You only mark your "best guess" if you are willing to bet $5 on it.
You only eliminate choices from guessing if you are willing to bet $5 on it.

Why $5? Five dollars is an amount of money that is small yet not insignificant, and can really add up fast (20 questions could cost you $100). Likewise, each answer choice on one question of the test will have a small impact on your overall score, but it can really add up to a lot of points in the end.

The process of elimination IS valuable. The following shows your chance of guessing it right:

If you eliminate wrong answer choices until only this many answer choices remain:	1	2	3
Chance of getting it correct:	100%	50%	33%

However, if you accidentally eliminate the right answer or go on a hunch for an incorrect answer, your chances drop dramatically: to 0%. By guessing among all the answer choices, you are GUARANTEED to have a shot at the right answer.

That's why the $5 test is so valuable- if you give up the advantage and safety of a pure guess, it had better be worth the risk.

What we still haven't covered is how to be sure that whatever guess you make is truly random. Here's the easiest way:

Always pick the first answer choice among those remaining.

Such a technique means that you have decided, **before you see a single test question**, exactly how you are going to guess- and since the order of choices tells you nothing about which one is correct, this guessing technique is perfectly random.

This section is not meant to scare you away from making educated guesses or eliminating choices- you just need to define when a choice is worth eliminating. The $5 test, along with a pre-defined random guessing strategy, is the best way to make sure you reap all of the benefits of guessing.

Secret Key #3 - Practice Smarter, Not Harder

Many test takers delay the test preparation process because they dread the awful amounts of practice time they think necessary to succeed on the test. We have refined an effective method that will take you only a fraction of the time.

There are a number of "obstacles" in your way to succeed. Among these are answering questions, finishing in time, and mastering test-taking strategies. All must be executed on the day of the test at peak performance, or your score will suffer. The test is a mental marathon that has a large impact on your future.

Just like a marathon runner, it is important to work your way up to the full challenge. So first you just worry about questions, and then time, and finally strategy:

Success Strategy

1. Find a good source for practice tests.
2. If you are willing to make a larger time investment, consider using more than one study guide- often the different approaches of multiple authors will help you "get" difficult concepts.
3. Take a practice test with no time constraints, with all study helps "open book." Take your time with questions and focus on applying strategies.
4. Take a practice test with time constraints, with all guides "open book."
5. Take a final practice test with no open material and time limits

If you have time to take more practice tests, just repeat step 5. By gradually exposing yourself to the full rigors of the test environment, you will condition your mind to the stress of test day and maximize your success.

Secret Key #4 - Prepare, Don't Procrastinate

Let me state an obvious fact: if you take the test three times, you will get three different scores. This is due to the way you feel on test day, the level of preparedness you have, and, despite the test writers' claims to the contrary, some tests WILL be easier for you than others.

Since your future depends so much on your score, you should maximize your chances of success. In order to maximize the likelihood of success, you've got to prepare in advance. This means taking practice tests and spending time learning the information and test taking strategies you will need to succeed.

Never take the test as a "practice" test, expecting that you can just take it again if you need to. Feel free to take sample tests on your own, but when you go to take the official test, be prepared, be focused, and do your best the first time!

Secret Key #5 - Test Yourself

Everyone knows that time is money. There is no need to spend too much of your time or too little of your time preparing for the test. You should only spend as much of your precious time preparing as is necessary for you to get the score you need.

Once you have taken a practice test under real conditions of time constraints, then you will know if you are ready for the test or not.

If you have scored extremely high the first time that you take the practice test, then there is not much point in spending countless hours studying. You are already there.

Benchmark your abilities by retaking practice tests and seeing how much you have improved. Once you score high enough to guarantee success, then you are ready.

If you have scored well below where you need, then knuckle down and begin studying in earnest. Check your improvement regularly through the use of practice tests under real conditions. Above all, don't worry, panic, or give up. The key is perseverance!

Then, when you go to take the test, remain confident and remember how well you did on the practice tests. If you can score high enough on a practice test, then you can do the same on the real thing.

General Strategies

The most important thing you can do is to ignore your fears and jump into the test immediately- do not be overwhelmed by any strange-sounding terms. You have to jump into the test like jumping into a pool- all at once is the easiest way.

Make Predictions
As you read and understand the question, try to guess what the answer will be. Remember that several of the answer choices are wrong, and once you begin reading them, your mind will immediately become cluttered with answer choices designed to throw you off. Your mind is typically the most focused immediately after you have read the question and digested its contents. If you can, try to predict what the correct answer will be. You may be surprised at what you can predict.

Quickly scan the choices and see if your prediction is in the listed answer choices. If it is, then you can be quite confident that you have the right answer. It still won't hurt to check the other answer choices, but most of the time, you've got it!

Answer the Question
It may seem obvious to only pick answer choices that answer the question, but the test writers can create some excellent answer choices that are wrong. Don't pick an answer just because it sounds right, or you believe it to be true. It MUST answer the question. Once you've made your selection, always go back and check it against the question and make sure that you didn't misread the question, and the answer choice does answer the question posed.

Benchmark
After you read the first answer choice, decide if you think it sounds correct or not. If it doesn't, move on to the next answer choice. If it does, mentally mark that answer choice. This doesn't mean that you've definitely selected it as your answer choice, it just means that it's the best you've seen thus far. Go ahead and read the next choice. If the next choice is worse than the one you've already selected, keep going to the next answer choice. If the next choice is better than the choice you've already selected, mentally mark the new answer choice as your best guess.

The first answer choice that you select becomes your standard. Every other answer choice must be benchmarked against that standard. That choice is correct until proven otherwise by another answer choice beating it out. Once you've decided that no other answer choice seems as good, do one final check to ensure that your answer choice answers the question posed.

Valid Information
Don't discount any of the information provided in the question. Every piece of information may be necessary to determine the correct answer. None of the

information in the question is there to throw you off (while the answer choices will certainly have information to throw you off). If two seemingly unrelated topics are discussed, don't ignore either. You can be confident there is a relationship, or it wouldn't be included in the question, and you are probably going to have to determine what is that relationship to find the answer.

Avoid "Fact Traps"
Don't get distracted by a choice that is factually true. Your search is for the answer that answers the question. Stay focused and don't fall for an answer that is true but incorrect. Always go back to the question and make sure you're choosing an answer that actually answers the question and is not just a true statement. An answer can be factually correct, but it MUST answer the question asked. Additionally, two answers can both be seemingly correct, so be sure to read all of the answer choices, and make sure that you get the one that BEST answers the question.

Milk the Question
Some of the questions may throw you completely off. They might deal with a subject you have not been exposed to, or one that you haven't reviewed in years. While your lack of knowledge about the subject will be a hindrance, the question itself can give you many clues that will help you find the correct answer. Read the question carefully and look for clues. Watch particularly for adjectives and nouns describing difficult terms or words that you don't recognize. Regardless of if you completely understand a word or not, replacing it with a synonym either provided or one you more familiar with may help you to understand what the questions are asking. Rather than wracking your mind about specific detailed information concerning a difficult term or word, try to use mental substitutes that are easier to understand.

The Trap of Familiarity
Don't just choose a word because you recognize it. On difficult questions, you may not recognize a number of words in the answer choices. The test writers don't put "make-believe" words on the test; so don't think that just because you only recognize all the words in one answer choice means that answer choice must be correct. If you only recognize words in one answer choice, then focus on that one. Is it correct? Try your best to determine if it is correct. If it is, that is great, but if it doesn't, eliminate it. Each word and answer choice you eliminate increases your chances of getting the question correct, even if you then have to guess among the unfamiliar choices.

Eliminate Answers
Eliminate choices as soon as you realize they are wrong. But be careful! Make sure you consider all of the possible answer choices. Just because one appears right, doesn't mean that the next one won't be even better! The test writers will usually put more than one good answer choice for every question, so read all of them. Don't worry if you are stuck between two that seem right. By getting down to just two

remaining possible choices, your odds are now 50/50. Rather than wasting too much time, play the odds. You are guessing, but guessing wisely, because you've been able to knock out some of the answer choices that you know are wrong. If you are eliminating choices and realize that the last answer choice you are left with is also obviously wrong, don't panic. Start over and consider each choice again. There may easily be something that you missed the first time and will realize on the second pass.

Tough Questions
If you are stumped on a problem or it appears too hard or too difficult, don't waste time. Move on! Remember though, if you can quickly check for obviously incorrect answer choices, your chances of guessing correctly are greatly improved. Before you completely give up, at least try to knock out a couple of possible answers. Eliminate what you can and then guess at the remaining answer choices before moving on.

Brainstorm
If you get stuck on a difficult question, spend a few seconds quickly brainstorming. Run through the complete list of possible answer choices. Look at each choice and ask yourself, "Could this answer the question satisfactorily?" Go through each answer choice and consider it independently of the other. By systematically going through all possibilities, you may find something that you would otherwise overlook. Remember that when you get stuck, it's important to try to keep moving.

Read Carefully
Understand the problem. Read the question and answer choices carefully. Don't miss the question because you misread the terms. You have plenty of time to read each question thoroughly and make sure you understand what is being asked. Yet a happy medium must be attained, so don't waste too much time. You must read carefully, but efficiently.

Face Value
When in doubt, use common sense. Always accept the situation in the problem at face value. Don't read too much into it. These problems will not require you to make huge leaps of logic. The test writers aren't trying to throw you off with a cheap trick. If you have to go beyond creativity and make a leap of logic in order to have an answer choice answer the question, then you should look at the other answer choices. Don't overcomplicate the problem by creating theoretical relationships or explanations that will warp time or space. These are normal problems rooted in reality. It's just that the applicable relationship or explanation may not be readily apparent and you have to figure things out. Use your common sense to interpret anything that isn't clear.

Prefixes
If you're having trouble with a word in the question or answer choices, try

dissecting it. Take advantage of every clue that the word might include. Prefixes and suffixes can be a huge help. Usually they allow you to determine a basic meaning. Pre- means before, post- means after, pro - is positive, de- is negative. From these prefixes and suffixes, you can get an idea of the general meaning of the word and try to put it into context. Beware though of any traps. Just because con is the opposite of pro, doesn't necessarily mean congress is the opposite of progress!

Hedge Phrases
Watch out for critical "hedge" phrases, such as likely, may, can, will often, sometimes, often, almost, mostly, usually, generally, rarely, sometimes. Question writers insert these hedge phrases to cover every possibility. Often an answer choice will be wrong simply because it leaves no room for exception. Avoid answer choices that have definitive words like "exactly," and "always".

Switchback Words
Stay alert for "switchbacks". These are the words and phrases frequently used to alert you to shifts in thought. The most common switchback word is "but". Others include although, however, nevertheless, on the other hand, even though, while, in spite of, despite, regardless of.

New Information
Correct answer choices will rarely have completely new information included. Answer choices typically are straightforward reflections of the material asked about and will directly relate to the question. If a new piece of information is included in an answer choice that doesn't even seem to relate to the topic being asked about, then that answer choice is likely incorrect. All of the information needed to answer the question is usually provided for you, and so you should not have to make guesses that are unsupported or choose answer choices that require unknown information that cannot be reasoned on its own.

Time Management
On technical questions, don't get lost on the technical terms. Don't spend too much time on any one question. If you don't know what a term means, then since you don't have a dictionary, odds are you aren't going to get much further. You should immediately recognize terms as whether or not you know them. If you don't, work with the other clues that you have, the other answer choices and terms provided, but don't waste too much time trying to figure out a difficult term.

Contextual Clues
Look for contextual clues. An answer can be right but not correct. The contextual clues will help you find the answer that is most right and is correct. Understand the context in which a phrase or statement is made. This will help you make important distinctions.

Don't Panic
Panicking will not answer any questions for you. Therefore, it isn't helpful. When you first see the question, if your mind goes blank, take a deep breath. Force yourself to mechanically go through the steps of solving the problem and using the strategies you've learned.

Pace Yourself
Don't get clock fever. It's easy to be overwhelmed when you're looking at a page full of questions, your mind is full of random thoughts and feeling confused, and the clock is ticking down faster than you would like. Calm down and maintain the pace that you have set for yourself. As long as you are on track by monitoring your pace, you are guaranteed to have enough time for yourself. When you get to the last few minutes of the test, it may seem like you won't have enough time left, but if you only have as many questions as you should have left at that point, then you're right on track!

Answer Selection
The best way to pick an answer choice is to eliminate all of those that are wrong, until only one is left and confirm that is the correct answer. Sometimes though, an answer choice may immediately look right. Be careful! Take a second to make sure that the other choices are not equally obvious. Don't make a hasty mistake. There are only two times that you should stop before checking other answers. First is when you are positive that the answer choice you have selected is correct. Second is when time is almost out and you have to make a quick guess!

Check Your Work
Since you will probably not know every term listed and the answer to every question, it is important that you get credit for the ones that you do know. Don't miss any questions through careless mistakes. If at all possible, try to take a second to look back over your answer selection and make sure you've selected the correct answer choice and haven't made a costly careless mistake (such as marking an answer choice that you didn't mean to mark). This quick double check should more than pay for itself in caught mistakes for the time it costs.

Beware of Directly Quoted Answers
Sometimes an answer choice will repeat word for word a portion of the question or reference section. However, beware of such exact duplication – it may be a trap! More than likely, the correct choice will paraphrase or summarize a point, rather than being exactly the same wording.

Slang
Scientific sounding answers are better than slang ones. An answer choice that begins "To compare the outcomes..." is much more likely to be correct than one that begins "Because some people insisted..."

Extreme Statements

Avoid wild answers that throw out highly controversial ideas that are proclaimed as established fact. An answer choice that states the "process should be used in certain situations, if..." is much more likely to be correct than one that states the "process should be discontinued completely." The first is a calm rational statement and doesn't even make a definitive, uncompromising stance, using a hedge word "if" to provide wiggle room, whereas the second choice is a radical idea and far more extreme.

Answer Choice Families

When you have two or more answer choices that are direct opposites or parallels, one of them is usually the correct answer. For instance, if one answer choice states "x increases" and another answer choice states "x decreases" or "y increases," then those two or three answer choices are very similar in construction and fall into the same family of answer choices. A family of answer choices is when two or three answer choices are very similar in construction, and yet often have a directly opposite meaning. Usually the correct answer choice will be in that family of answer choices. The "odd man out" or answer choice that doesn't seem to fit the parallel construction of the other answer choices is more likely to be incorrect.

Be Aware of the Following Hints

National Board Dental Examination Part I

Sign-in	Tutorial
3.5 hours	Randomly-ordered, discipline-based test items 6-8 testlets (approximately 200 items)
Optional lunch break	Maximum one hour
3.5 hours	Randomly-ordered, discipline-based test items 6-8 testlets (approximately 200 items)

Registering for the NBDE Part I Licensure Test

Contact Information

The Joint Commission on National Dental Examinations
American Dental Association
211 East Chicago Avenue, 6th Floor
Chicago, Ill 60611
(312) 440-2678
http://www.ada.org

http://www.ada.org

Paper Test Registration Information:
Registration Deadline   **Test Date**
June 7, 2004   July 12, 2004
November 1, 2004   December 13, 2004

Exam Content

NBDE Part I Score Reporting

There is no penalty for guessing on the the NBDE Part I. A candidate's total score is reported in terms of a standard score, which has been converted from the total number of correct answers.

Special Report- Study Guides and Practice Tests Are Worth Your Time

We believe the following practice tests and guide present uncommon value to our customers who wish to "really study" for the NBDE Part I tests. While our manual teaches some valuable tricks and tips that no one else covers, learning the basic coursework tested on the exam is also necessary.

Practice Questions

Practice Questions
http://www.kaptest.com/Dental/NBDE/View-Kaplan-Programs/Online-Programs/DN_nbde_qbank1.html

Study Guides

National Dental Boards (Admission Test Series, Part 1)
http://www.amazon.com/exec/obidos/tg/detail/-/083736955X/qid=1085600857/sr=8-7/ref=sr_8_xs_ap_i7_xgl14/102-0090207-1636132?v=glance&s=books&n=507846

Review of Basic Science and Clinical Dentistry: Basic Science
http://www.amazon.com/exec/obidos/tg/detail/-/1550092006/ref=pd_bxgy_text_1/102-0090207-1636132?v=glance&s=books&st=*

These guides are THE best comprehensive coursework guides to the licensure exams. If you want to spend a couple months in preparation to squeeze every last drop out of your score, buy these books!

Special Report– Quick Reference Lesion Review

Occipital Lobe	Homonymous hemianopsia, partial seizures with limited visual phenomena
Thalamus	Contralateral thalamus pain, contralateral hemisensory loss
Pineal gland	Early hydrocephalus, papillary abnormalities, Parinaud's syndrome
Internal capsule	Hemisensory loss, homonymous hemianopsia, contralateral hemiplegia
Basal ganglia	Contralateral dystonia, Contralateral choreoathetosis
Pons	Diplopia, internal strabismus, VI and VII involvement, contralateral hemisensory and hemiparesis loss
Broca's area	Motor dysphasia
Precentral gyrus	Jacksonian seizures, generalized seizures, hemiparesis
Superficial parietal lobe	Receptive dysphasia
Cerebellar hemisphere	Ipsilateral cerebellar ataxia with hypotonia, dysmetria, intention tremor, nystagmus to side of lesion
Midbrain	Loss of upward gaze, III involvement, ipsilateral cerebellar signs, diplopia
Angular gyrus	Finger agnosia, allochiria, agraphia, acalculia
Temporal lobe	Contralateral homonymous upper quadrantanopsia, partial complex seizures
Paracentral lobe	Urgency of micturition, incontinence, progressive spastic paraparesis
Third Ventricle	Hydrocephalus
Fourth Ventricle	Hydrocephalus, progressive spastic hemiparesis
Optic Chiasm	Bitemporal hemianopsia, optic atrophy
Uncus	Partial complex seizures
Superior temporal gyrus	Receptive dysphasia
Prefrontal area	Apathy, poor attention span, loss of judgement, release phenomena, distractible
Orbital surface frontal lobe	Paroxysmal atrial tachycardia
Hypothalmus	Amenorrhea, cachexia, hypopituitarism, hypothyrodism, impotence, diencephalic

	autonomic seizures

Special Report- Review Tables and Images

Eruption Dates for Permanent Teeth

Tooth	Lower	Upper
Central Incisor	6 - 7 years	7 - 8 years
Lateral Incisor	7 - 8 years	8 - 9 years
Canine	9 - 10 years	11 - 12 years
1st Premolar	10 - 12 years	10 -11 years
2nd Premolar	11 - 12 years	10 - 12 years
1st Molar	6 - 7 years	6 - 7 years
2nd Molar	11 - 13 years	12 - 13 years
3rd Molar	17 - 21 years	17 - 21 years

Baby Teeth Eruption Dates

Tooth	Lower	Upper
Central Incisor	6 1/2 months	7 1/2 months
Lateral Incisor	7 months	8 months
First Molar	12 - 16 months	12 - 16 months
Canine	16 - 20 months	16 - 20 months
Second Molar	20 - 30 months	20 - 30 months

UPPER TEETH	ERUPT
Central Incisor	7-8 years
Lateral Incisor	8-9 years
Canine (Cuspid)	11-12 years
First Premolar (First Bicuspid)	10-11 years
Second Premolar (Second Bicuspid)	10-12 years
First Molar	6-7 years
Second Premolar	12-13 years
Third Molar (Wisdom Teeth)	17-21 years

LOWER TEETH	ERUPT
Third Molar (Wisdom Teeth)	17-21 years
Second Premolar	11-13 years
First Molar	6-7 years
Second Premolar (Second Bicuspid)	11-12 years
First Premolar (First Bicuspid)	10-12 years
Canine (Cuspid)	9-10 years
Lateral Incisor	7-8 years
Central Incisor	6-7 years

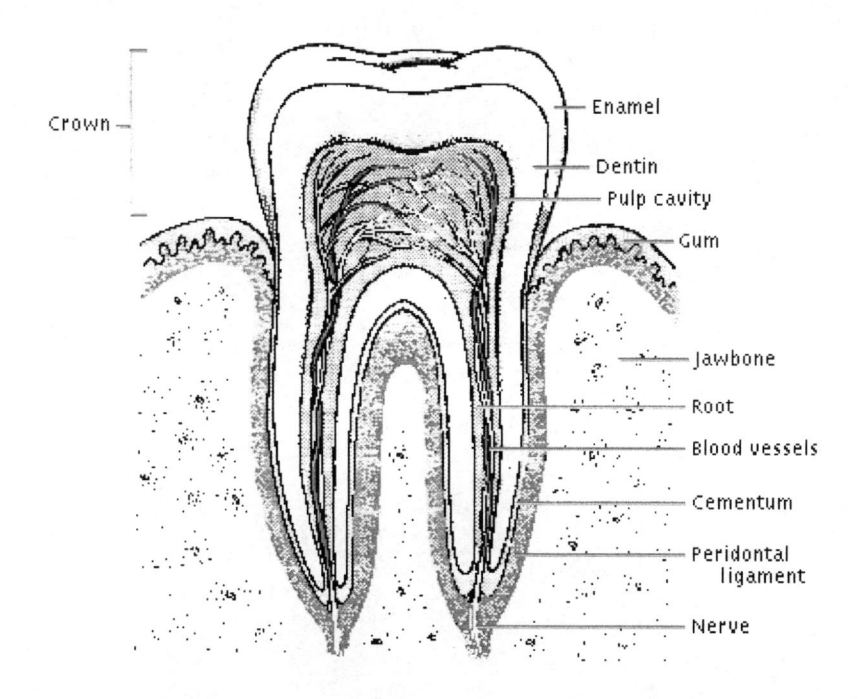

Lateral View

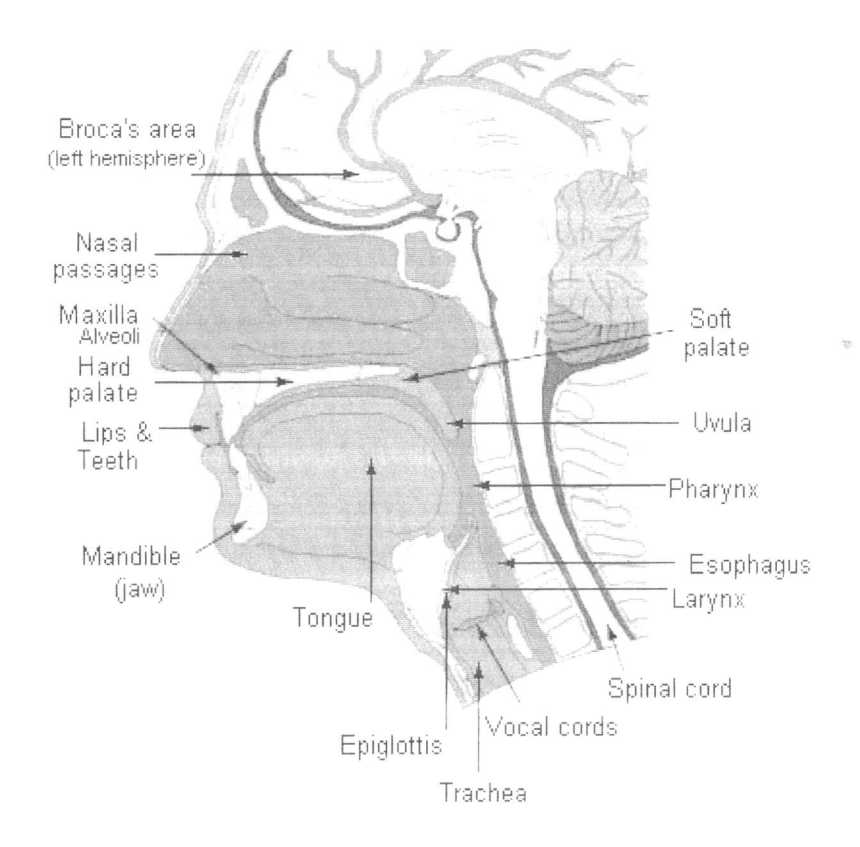

Skull Anatomy

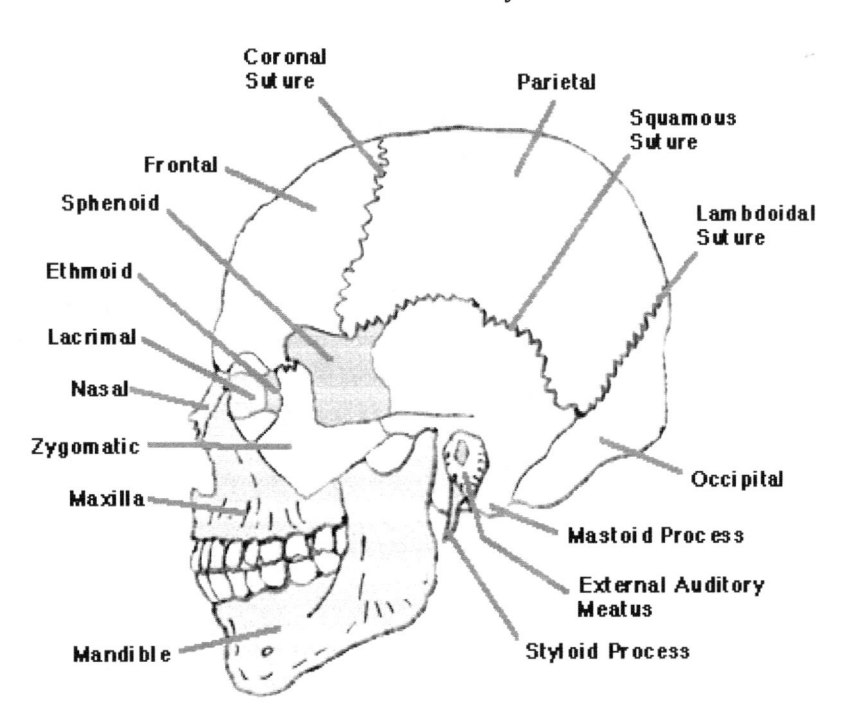

S.mutans Role in Plaque Formation

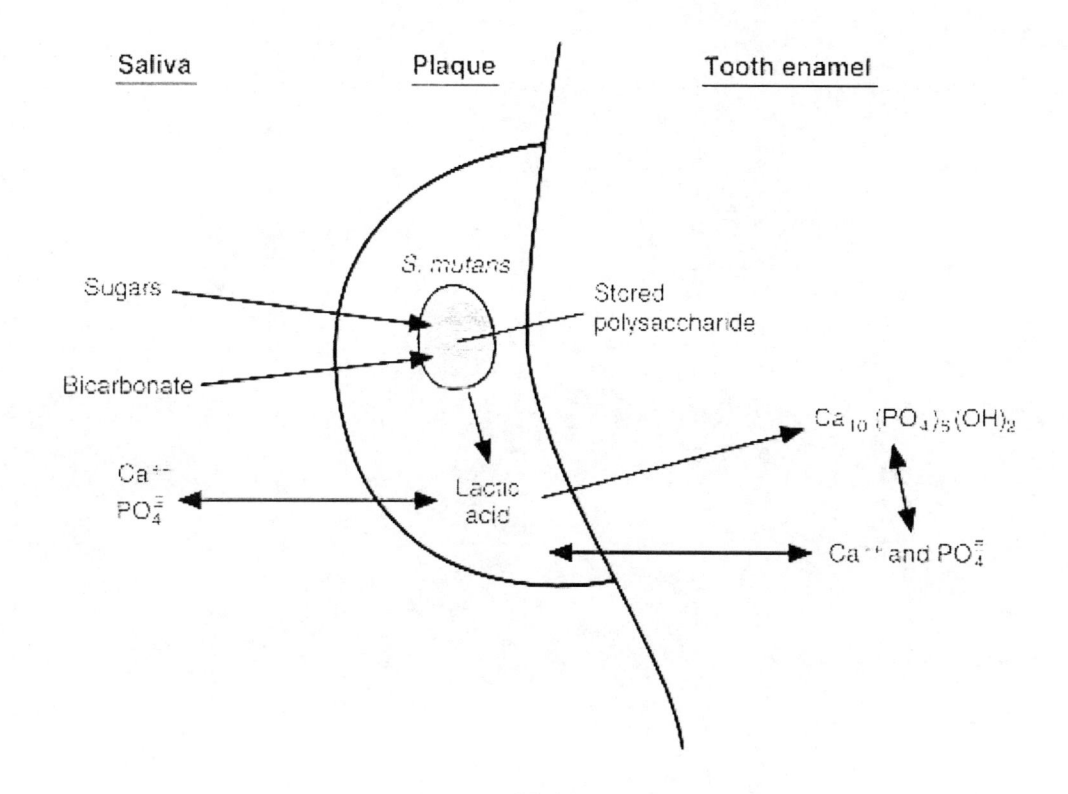

Saliva	Plaque	Tooth enamel

- Sugars → S. mutans
- Bicarbonate → S. mutans
- Stored polysaccharide
- S. mutans → Lactic acid
- Ca^{++}, $PO_4^{\equiv}$ ↔ Lactic acid
- Lactic acid → $Ca_{10}(PO_4)_6(OH)_2$ ↔ Ca^{++} and $PO_4^{\equiv}$

Role of Fluoride

1. Tooth mineral is made less soluble by the formation of fluorapatite during development

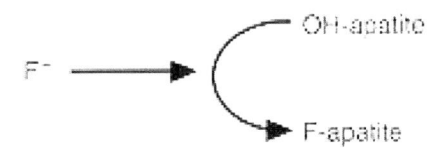

F^- → OH-apatite → F-apatite

2. Fluoride in saliva and plaque promotes remineralization of tooth surface after tooth eruption

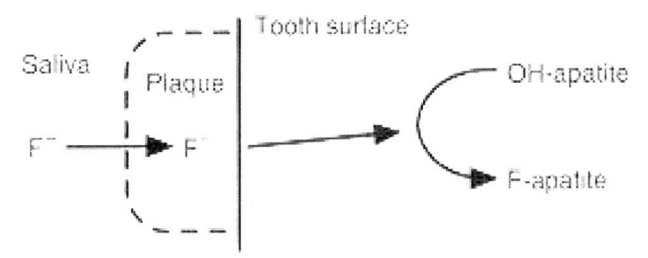

Saliva F^- → Plaque F^- → Tooth surface: OH-apatite → F-apatite

3. Fluoride in plaque enters bacterial cells, especially at low pH, and inhibits enolase, thereby reducing acid production in plaque

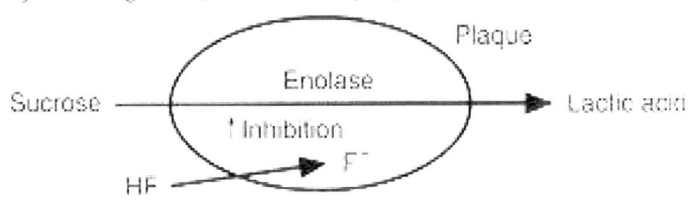

Plaque: Sucrose → (Enolase, ↑Inhibition by F^- from HF) → Lactic acid

Bonus Report – Dental Organizations

Academy for Sports Dentistry - Organization providing info and ideas for protection from sports related mouth injuries.

Academy of General Dentistry - Organization Committed to ongoing continuing education for Dentists.

Academy of Interdisciplinary Dentofacial Therapy - A comprehensive approach to patient care.

Academy of Laser Dentistry - Organization committed to laser education and research in Dentistry.

Academy of Osseointegration - Organization committed to furthering the education and research concerning implant dentistry.

Alpha Omega International Dental Fraternity - International group offering lectures, study groups, continuing education.

American Academy of Cosmetic Dentistry - Dedicated to advancing the Art and Science of Cosmetic Dentistry.

American Academy of Dental Hygiene - Fostering education and research in the field of dental hygiene.

American Academy of Dental Practice Administration - Committed to providing practice management information for dentists.

American Academy of Esthetic Dentistry - Promoting the integration of esthetics into the total spectrum of oral health care.

American Academy of Fixed Prosthodontics - Committed to competency in research and practice of crown and bridge prosthodontics.

American Academy of Implant Dentistry - Advancing the practice of Implant Dentistry through education and credentialing.

American Academy of Implant Prosthodontics - Providing ongoing training and support for excellence in Implant Dentistry.

American Academy of Maxillofacial Prosthetics - Dedicated to prosthetic correction and management of maxillofacial defects.

American Academy of Orofacial Pain - Includes a detailed tutorial about TMD and orofacial pain.

American Academy of Pediatric Dentistry - Oral health care for infants, children and adolescents.

American Academy of Periodontology - Committed to advancing the periodontal health of the public.

American Academy of Restorative Dentistry - The mission of the Academy is to promote the improvement of the health of the public, and the quality of the art and science of restorative dentistry.

American Association for Dental Research - To represent and support the oral health research community.

American Association for Dental Research - Chicago Section - An organization committed to supporting dental research..

American Association of Dental Schools - All U.S. and Canadian Dental Schools and continuing education programs.
American Association of Endodontists - Promoting research and ideas to encourage excellence in endodontics.
American Association of Oral and Maxillofacial Surgeons - Organization of maxillofacial surgeons.
American Association of Oral Biologists - An independent association supporting education, research and clinical practice in the discipline of Oral Biology.
American Association of Orthodontists - Association committed to educating the public and advancing the art of orthodontics.
American Association of Public Health Dentistry - Supporting and promoting public education and awareness of oral health care.
American Board of Forensic Odontology - The Board that sets the standards for dentists practicing forensic odontology.
American Cleft Palate-Craniofacial Association - Research and education for specialists and families of individuals with cleft palate.
American College of Dentists - Organization of leaders in Dentistry who have made major contributions to dentistry.
American College of Forensic Examiners - Providing education and training for forensic examinations.
American College of Prosthodontics - Promoting the high quality care of prosthodontic patients.
American Dental Assistants Association - To promote the dental assisting profession and promote education and legislation to enhance the delivery of quality denatl health care.
American Dental Association - The ADA is the leading dental site for professionals and consumer info.
American Dental Hygienists Association - Providing info to hygienists and to the public.
American Dental Society of Anesthesiology - Organization committed to education and high standards for anesthesiology and pain control.

Bonus Report – Guidelines for Universal Precautions

Universal precautions are precautions taken to avoid contracting various diseases and preventing the spread of disease to those who have compromised immunity. Some of these diseases include human immunodeficiency virus (HIV), acquired immunodeficiency syndrome (AIDS), and hepatitis B (HBV). Universal precautions are needed since many diseases do not display signs or symptoms in their early stages. Universal precautions mean to treat all body fluids/ substances as if they were contaminated. These body fluids include but are not limited to the following blood, semen, vaginal secretions, breast milk, amniotic fluid, feces, urine, peritoneal fluid, synovial fluid, cerebrospinal fluid, secretions from the nasal and oral cavities, and lacrimal and sweat gland excretions. This means that universal precautions should be used with all patients.

1. A shield for the eyes and face must be used if there is a possibility of splashes from blood and body fluids.
2. If possibility of blood or body fluids being splashed on clothing, you must wear a plastic apron.
3. Gloves must be worn if you could possibly come in contact with blood or body fluids. They are also needed if you are going to touch something that may have come in contact with blood or body fluids.
4. Hands must be washed even if you were wearing gloves. Hands must be washed and gloves must be changed between patients. Wash hands with at a dime size amount of soap and warm water for about 30 seconds. Singing "Mary had a little lamb" is approximately 30 seconds.
5. Blood and body fluid spills must be cleansed and disinfected using a solution of one part bleach to 10 parts water or your hospital's accepted method.
6. Used needles must be separated from clean needles. Throw both the needle and the syringe away in the sharps' container. The sharps' container is made of puncture proof material.
7. Take extra care in performing high-risk activities that include puncturing the skin and cutting the skin.
8. CPR equipment to be used in a hospital must include resuscitation bags and mouthpieces.

Special precautions must be taken to dispose of biomedical waste. Biomedical waste includes but is not limited to the following: laboratory waste, pathology waste, liquid waste from suction, all sharp object, bladder catheters, chest tubes, IV tubes, and drainage containers. Biomedical waste is removed from a facility by trained biomedical waste disposers.

The health care professional is legally and ethically responsible for adhering to universal precautions. They may prevent you from contracting a fatal disease or from a patient contracting a disease from you that could be deadly.

CPR Review/Cheat Sheet

Topic	New Guidelines
Conscious Choking	5 back blows, then 5 abdominal thrusts- adult/child
Unconscious Choking	5 chest compressions, look, 2 breaths-adult/child/infant
Rescue Breaths	Normal Breath given over 1 second until chest rises
Chest Compressions to Ventilation Ratios (Single Rescuer)	30:2 – Adult/Child/Infant
Chest Compressions to Ventilation Ratios (Two Rescuer)	30:2 – Adult 15:2 – Child/Infant
Chest Compression rate	About 100/minute – Adult/Child/Infant
Chest Compression Land marking Method	Simplified approach – center of the chest – Adult/Child 2 or 3 fingers, just below the nipple line at the center of the chest - Infant
AED	1 shock, then 2 minutes (or 5 cycles) of CPR
Anaphylaxis	Assist person with use of prescribed auto injector
Asthma	Assist person with use of prescribed inhaler

- Check the scene
- Check for responsiveness – ask, "Are you OK?"
- Adult - call 911, then administer CPR
- Child/Infant – administer CPR for 5 cycles, then call 911
- Open victim's airway and check for breathing – look, listen, and feel for 5 - 10 seconds
- Two rescue breaths should be given, 1 second each, and should produce a visible chest rise
- If the air does not go in, reposition and try 2 breaths again
- Check victim's pulse – chest compressions are recommended if an infant or child has a rate less than 60 per minute with signs of poor perfusion.
- Begin 30 compressions to 2 breaths at a rate of 1 breath every 5 seconds for Adult; 1 breath every 3 seconds for child/infant
- Continue 30:2 ratio until victim moves, AED is brought to the scene, or professional help arrives

AED

- ADULT/ Child over 8 years old - use Adult pads
- Child 1-8 years old – use Child pads or use Adult pads by placing one on the chest and one on the back of the child
- Infant under 1 year of age - AED not recommended